STATE OF BLACK LOUISVILLE

2 0 1 8 R E P O R T

ACKNOWLEDGMENTS

We gratefully acknowledge the many contributors to this project. It would not have been possible without the continued support of our partners, colleagues and donors. We want to express our deepest appreciation to those who donated time and services.

EXECUTIVE EDITOR
Ashli Findley

ASSOCIATE EDITOR
Sadiqa Reynolds

COPY EDITORS
Ashli Findley
Sadiqa Reynolds
Lyndon Pryor

CONTRIBUTORS
Dr. Anita P. Barbee; Brian C.B. Barnes; Dr. Matt Berry; Dr. Craig Blakely; Shandelier Boyd Smith; Dorian O. Burton; Dr. Karan Chavis; Dr. Kevin Cosby; Kevin Cowherd; Raoul Cunningham; Jennie Jean Davidson; Dr. Cherie Dawson-Edwards; Hannah Drake; Kevin Dunlap; Timothy E. Findley, Jr.; Ted Gatlin, Jr.; Yvette Gentry; Chanelle Helm; Dr. Vicki P. Hines-Martin; Cathy Hinko; Alicia Hurle; Bill Huston; Dana Jackson; Nikki R. Jackson; Dr. Ricky L. Jones; Virginia Kelly Judd; Dr. Brandy N. Kelly Pryor; Harrison Kirby; Dr. Bertis Little; Jessica Lucas; Dr. John Marshall; Carolyn Miller-Cooper (deceased); Mary Montgomery; Karyn Moskowitz; Sharon Murphy; Gisela Nelson; Dr. Armon R. Perry; Joshua Poe; Lyndon Pryor; Ben Reno-Weber; Theresa Reno-Weber; Sadiqa Reynolds, Esq.; "SCZ"; Anthony Smith; Lisa Thompson; Daryle Unseld Jr.; Dr. Ahmad Washington; Mary Gwen Wheeler; Dr. F. Bruce Williams; LaGraica Williams; Betty Winston Baye'

ARTISTS
Marc Murphy
Carey Payne

BOARD OF DIRECTORS
Lorri Lee--Board Chair; Mike Bellissimo; Neville Blakemore; James Calleroz White, PhD; Condrad Daniels; Sharon Decker; Jorge De La Jara; Trisha Finnegan; Ted Gatlin, Jr.; Hood Harris; Dwight Haygood, Jr.; Hunt Helm; Earl Jones; Walter Koczot; Terryl McCray; Ryan P. Parker; A. Diane Porter; Wooford R. Porter, Jr.; Nancy Presnell; Stephen Reily; A. Ben Ruiz; Doug Smith; Neal Thomas

CONTENTS

HEALTH

HOUSING

REFERENCES AND DATA

Louisville Urban League

THE LOUISVILLE URBAN LEAGUE is a nonprofit, nonpartisan, community service organization dedicated to eliminating racism and its adverse impacts on our community. Our mission is to assist African Americans and other marginalized populations in attaining social and economic equality through direct services and advocacy in the areas of education, employment, housing, family development, and community development.

In 1920, just 10 years after what would become the National Urban League, the Louisville Urban League was founded and became a member agency of the local Community Chest. Elwood Street, serving as temporary chairman, appointed a five-person committee to create the framework for the local Urban League. The agency started with $1,000 raised by community residents at a public dinner. Incorporated in August 1921, the Urban League of Louisville for Social Service Among Negroes eventually became the Louisville Urban League.

The leadership of the Louisville Urban League developed a strategic plan to create and nurture enduring relationships between the League, community leaders, public officials, and the business sector. In fact, the Louisville Urban League is the oldest HUD-certified housing counseling agency in the Commonwealth of Kentucky.

For nearly 100 years, the Louisville Urban League has been a consistent voice and a liaison for the city's underserved and minority populations. It will continue to address current issues and challenges with steadfast and sustainable solutions through direct services and advocacy in the areas of Jobs, Justice, Education, Health and Housing.

EXECUTIVE SUMMARY

Ashli Findley, Editor

The State of Black Louisville 2018 is a collection of essays from engaged stakeholders, presenting the state of affairs of African Americans in the areas of jobs, justice, education, health, and housing. Leading figures and field experts from the Louisville community have furnished the report with data, benchmarks, insightful analysis, reflective commentary, and thought leadership around both the disparities and improvements that African Americans face in these areas. Each essay also provides recommendations and solutions-oriented action items.

We have anticipated the release of the report. Not only does it provides a clear and accurate picture of the livelihood of African Americans living in Louisville, but it also presents a strong call to action to move policy forward that would have far-reaching impact. The advancement of the ideas and ideals echoed throughout this report will take all of us working together – from legislators to lay residents. The saying, "I did not know" is no longer valid.

As we push for a more equitable Louisville, let us also recognize that this year is the 50th anniversary of the Poor People's march on Washington, spawned by Dr. Martin Luther King Jr., and his Poor People's Campaign. The purpose of the march was to demand better jobs, better homes, and better education for the poor of all races. Dr. King sought to have basic questions answered about our society and government, namely the root causes of economic disparity, with a call for redistribution of economic and political power.

The initial gathering of leadership joining the campaign included representation from over fifty multiracial, societal organizations. Dr. King addressed the group, saying that it was the first meeting of that kind he had ever participated in.[1]

In similar fashion, the State of Black Louisville 2018 brings together leadership representation from multiple organizations across the Louisville community. They have joined to collectively address the harsh realities for many who call this city home, and to use their voice and platform to advance the change. We salute those who have and will continue the march for equality for all.

INTRODUCTION

Sadiqa Reynolds, Esq., President and CEO
Louisville Urban League

Imagine sitting down to a game of Monopoly. Everyone else at the table has been playing 400 years. Everyone but you. Still, you join the game. Of course, because you are late, by the time you start some players have acquired boatloads of money. Others have lost as much, but they all have had 400 years of experience learning the game, creating the rules, adjusting for flaws. These are all things that a new player would have to "catch up" on.

Now suppose only half the players want you in the game. The remainder resents your presence, your delay in participation, and constantly reminds you of how great the game was before you got in.

Where does the new player get the resources to join the game? Do you begin with the same amount of money as players who started 400 years ago? If so, how do you ever really exert any influence over the board? After all, most of the land is owned by others. Boardwalk is gone and many players own hotels all around the board. Every place you land, you must pay some sort of tax.

Each time you make it around the board you pay $200, just like every other player passing "Go." The challenge is that every payment comes close to bankrupting you. You've had no access to resources available to other players, because the rules were set before you got in. It gets to the point where landing on "Go to Jail" is the only space safe from the tax of life.

Your presence is felt because the time you take to learn the rules and roll the dice slows the game. You are constantly reminded that you can't be a serious player because there is no way you can ever really win.

The late player, the Black player, isn't playing Monopoly. The Black player is playing "Survival." A few of us get lucky and thrive, but most get caught in a system that we are ill-prepared to enter and within which our presence is resented.

It is incumbent upon us to remind ourselves and others that we are the only immigrants to this country brought in against our will and held entirely for the benefit of others. We are the descendants of slaves forced to immigrate into a country in which we are not responsible for our arrival and have had little to no say over our condition. Yet, we achieve in ways that were never imagined or intended, and quite often against all odds and in circumstances that would have broken a less-resilient people.

Our lack of wealth is not indicative of a lack of creativity, ideas, solutions, or effort. Power began to be acquired before the rules even allowed a seat at the table, a chance to play the game that's now 400 years old.

It's been a 400-year game. Two hundred and fifty years of slavery. Ninety years of Jim Crow. Sixty years of discriminatory housing policy. Countless examples of our presence being unwanted and our lives unvalued – and we are still here. The "Make America Great Again" slogan begs the question: Under what conditions do some have to live for America to be great, and for whom?

As we witness attacks on the gains that have been made, we also feel the hope of arriving at a crossroads and knowing that we have this moment to create new alliances and collaborations to push toward a world that reflects justice and equity rather than one that sets America back again.

We do not have the resources to significantly invest in our own communities. We can't self-fund large-scale capital projects. We can't even control the costs of necessities in the communities in which we live. Our investment needs require charity or, we would argue, justice.

We need intentional investment in the dreams of Black Americans and capital investment with Black ownership on the other side of that deal. White Americans have had the ability and resources to take risk, finding great success and, at times, great failure. Yet, society seems to attribute Black failure to ignorance or incompetence. We get one shot, by one

star, who we must pray doesn't choke. Should our star hit the shot, and the celebration ensues, we then pray they stay loyal to the movement even when the other team begins to recruit.

This pressure of being Black in America … Black in Louisville … is aspiration-crushing.

If America is ever to be great, she must tell the truth of the history of Black people in this country. She must constantly tell the truth that we did not arrive on this planet as slaves. She must change the misleading narrative playing about who and what Black people are and how she has benefited from keeping us in our place.

There can be no peace without justice and no justice without truth. In fact, Louisville must tell the truth of its history and begin to deal with the real effects of discrimination, redlining, bias, and dog whistles.

The challenges in our city are the same as those present for Black people in every city in this country. Access to capital is limited and, when it comes, it is directive and sparse. We are invited to the table as observers but not empowered to disagree or set our own course.

We are free to speak our minds but only to the extent that we understand our message could result in frustration on the part of those with the resources we desperately need. Sometimes other Blacks view those making it into the higher levels of the game as sellouts. Sadly, sometimes they are. However, many of us remain true in every room we enter and we are here fighting for change. Indeed, it is sometimes our presence that keeps all of us from being sold down river again.

So, in a sense, this report is our effort to … at a minimum … own our voices. Whatever the cost.

LOUISVILLE DOESN'T EVEN KNOW WHAT IT HAS STOLEN FROM BLACKS

Dr. Kevin Cosby, Pastor; President
St. Stephen Church
Simmons College of Kentucky

The problem for Blacks in America is not that we don't pray. Instead, we have been the prey of what President Lyndon Johnson referred to as "ancient brutalities, past injustice and present prejudice."[2]

I totally disagree with political pundits who argue that government "can't fix the problem" of Black America. To the contrary, only government has the resources to do so. Only government can prevent Black America from becoming our nation's permanent underclass. Although Blacks have been in America longer than almost every other ethnic group, we lag in every socio-economic measurement for progress. Black America is doing the worst, because for centuries Black America has endured the worst. No group has been legally restricted from full participation in the American dream. Today, Black people are still grappling with the consequences of legally-sanctioned, horrific and inhumane treatment.

The greatest myth that has been perpetuated in America in the last 50 years is that of how America became so racially segregated.

In every metropolitan area in America, there are poor, Black neighborhoods, like many of the neighborhoods in west Louisville. The common myth that most Americans hold is the misguided notion that segregated neighborhoods are the result of de facto segregation, which resulted from private prejudices against Blacks. It is falsely believed that private prejudices led to White flight and the effort to sustain all-White neighborhoods.

Such an interpretation absolves the government from intervention. Government has no constitutional right or obligation to remedy Black poverty because of de facto segregation. Separating oneself is within the right of every racist American, regardless of how objectionable we may find it today.

The idea that de facto segregation or personal

prejudice caused a segregated west Louisville and other poor, Black communities throughout America is a conventional myth. It allows politicians to feel justified in saying government has no role in addressing the societal ills of Black America. The plain, undeniable fact of history is that segregation in America is the consequence of de jure, or state-sponsored causes. Since slavery in America, federal, state and local governments have enacted unconstitutional public policies that have created the present racial divide.

The United States government engineered racially-segregated neighborhoods like west Louisville and created economic incentives for Whites to participate in it.

Public housing during the Great Depression and after World War II was legally segregated by government mandate. Housing complexes like Cabrini Green and Robert Taylor homes in Chicago were created for Blacks by the federal government because Blacks were barred from living in public housing created for Whites. Other practices, like redlining of mortgages, prevented economic investment in Black neighborhoods while providing FHA subsidies for builders on the basis that no homes in White neighborhoods be built for or sold to African-Americans.

The only reason White flight occurred after World War II is that the government created provisions for White flight and Black exclusion. Sprawling suburban neighborhoods like Levittown were built by the federal government on the basis that Blacks be excluded. Levitt homes were purchased by Whites at a discounted price. The White homeowners made minimal financial mortgage investments, but received maximum equity in their homes, which created wealth. While Whites were given these privileges, Blacks were kept out. In fact, Blacks were paying more for living in public housing than Whites were paying to own Levitt homes.

These government-sponsored, Whites-only housing complexes gave Whites home equity that Blacks were unable to accumulate. These and similar practices are the roots of the present-day wealth gap between Blacks and Whites. The average American's wealth is tied up in their home's equity. So, as White baby boomers are retiring and expiring, they are able to pass down to their children wealth from home equity that Black baby boomers were blocked from acquiring.

One of the greatest examples of how the government created segregated housing was right here in Louisville in 1954. An African-American couple, Andrew and Charlotte Wade, desired to purchase a home in Shively. Because it was an all-White community, a White couple, Carl and Anne Braden, had to purchase the house for them.

Andrew Wade was an electrical contractor and Korean War Navy veteran. The day he moved his family into his Shively home, a crowd gathered in front of his house to intimidate them. A cross was burned in front of his house. A rock was thrown through his window with a message tied to it, "Nigger get out!" For a whole month, demonstrations persisted outside his home. Eventually, their home was dynamited. These actions of terror and intimidation forced the Wades back to the segregated Black community.

No one was arrested for crimes related to this incident. That is, no one except Carl and Ann Braden. A grand jury indicted them on charges of sedition for stirring up racial conflict by selling a house to African-Americans. Carl Braden was sentenced to 15 years in prison. In his famous, "Letter From Birmingham Jail," Dr. Martin Luther King, Jr., pays tribute to Ann Braden for her courageous act of fighting state-sponsored segregation.

As a child growing up in west Louisville, I never understood why my parents never went to Shively, nor did they allow us to go. As a result of the Wade's experience, many Blacks never tried to move out of a segregated west Louisville until 1970. These actions by government just 60 years ago are a major reason we have poor, segregated neighborhoods in west Louisville today.

When segregation is the result of de facto causes, as tragic as it may be, the government has no constitutional remedies. But when the segregation is caused by the government, then the government has both a constitutional obligation and moral responsibility to remedy it.

The government violated the equal protection clause of the 14th Amendment. Now, government has to fix it. Rectifying these evils of our past will take more than prayer.

The process of remedy will begin with an acknowledgment of the years of legally-sanctioned segregation and how we are living with the consequences today. The biblical word for this is confession. After confession comes another biblical action called repentance. This level of remorse is more than saying, "I am sorry," rather, it is an attempt to reverse the evil course that public policies have initiated. For example, if you steal my car on Monday and get saved on Tuesday, yet you continue driving my car on Wednesday, then you weren't truly saved on Tuesday. The sign that you were truly saved on Tuesday is that you return my car to me on Wednesday.

The problem in Louisville is that our community does not even know what it has stolen from Blacks because this painful history has been suppressed in our memory. What is too painful to face we often seek to forget or ignore. Suppressing the memory will not suppress the consequences. These we see in west Louisville every day.

What elected officials should do is come to the Black community and offer an official apology for the atrocities the Commonwealth of Kentucky has committed against African-Americans in this state. Further, they should pledge to sensitize Whites to this dark chapter in our history and the effects it has on our present-day crisis. They should also relieve the Black community of the psychological burden we often feel for the shape of our community. Our problem is, like the Wade's, we have been preyed upon.

The governor should announce a governor's initiative to convene as many stakeholders as possible to study the root causes and cures for the problems that plague west Louisville and use that platform to marshal both private and public funds to remedy the destruction that government legislated in west Louisville and against Blacks across our state.

It was bad government that put Blacks in chains as slaves for 246 years and it took good government to end slavery. Bad government said in the Dred Scott Supreme Court decision that Blacks had no rights that Whites were bound to respect, and it took good government to correct it. It was bad government that legally segregated Blacks until the late 1960s, and it took good government to correct it. Bad government kept Blacks on the back of the bus, but good government made room for us on the front of the bus.

Bad government kept Blacks out of the University of Louisville and University of Kentucky, but good government opened those doors. Bad government kept Blacks from voting, but good government gave us the vote. Bad government has filled our jails and prisons with Black men with disproportionate sentences and it will take good government to fix it. Bad government created residential segregation, and it will take good government in 2017 and beyond to finally overcome it.

Blatant insensitivity simply reinforces stereotypes many have about Blacks. Political pandering takes advantage of White ignorance of our recent racist past and how that past has shaped our present.

More than anything, feigned attempts at offering real solutions cause severe pain to a community that is already hurting from being blamed for what *their* government has done.

What the Black community really needs is justice. Whites sometimes downplay the extent and the effects of racism. Blacks are accused of playing the race card and making mountains out of molehills. Whites often point to anecdotal evidence of Black progress in America through individual success stories like Oprah Winfrey, Michael Jordan, and Barack Obama.

Social critic Antonio Moore argues that Whites are often hypnotized by Black celebrity success which, in turn, desensitizes them to Black pain. Black celebrities have often successfully hidden from America the painful reality of mass Black suffering. Black wealth is sufficiently negligible to render it virtually non-existent. Black unemployment in most urban areas is 35 to 40% Black male incarceration exceeds the numbers of South Africa during apartheid.

Whites are often equally guilty of being ignorant about the privileges that come with Whiteness. Anti-racist activist George Lipsitz said, "Whiteness has cash value: it accounts for advantages that come to individuals through profits made from housing secured in discriminatory markets, through the unequal educational opportunities unavailable to children of different races, through insider networks that channel employment opportunities to relatives and friends of those who profited the most from present and past discrimination, especially through intergenerational transfers of inherited wealth that pass down the spoils of discrimination to succeeding generations."[3]

The greatest tragedy of Whites may be that they entangle the name of Christ with a movement that is connected to injustice. Just as Christ was used to justify slavery and Jim Crow, elected officials often put Christ on the side of anti-government intervention. This is one of the reasons why many thinking Black people are turned off by Christianity and call it a "White man's religion" or "Whitetianity."

It is time for the justice demands of the gospel to be realized.

Reprinted with permission from author.

YOU WERE BORN TO BE A PROBLEM...

Hannah Drake

In the Souls of Black Folk W.E.B. Dubois eloquently penned, "Between me and the other world there is ever an unasked question: unasked by some through feelings of delicacy; by others through the difficulty of rightly framing it. All, nevertheless, flutter round it, "How does it feel to be a problem?"
How does it feel not to just have a problem… but to be the problem?
That your very existence, the fact you are breathing air is problematic?
How does it feel to be a problem?

The usual suspect, murdered live on social media by those sworn to serve and protect, gunned down in the streets holding Skittles and tea, memorialized on Twitter with Rest in Peace shirts and hashtags all while they continue to fill out toetags?
How does it feel knowing that 32% of Black males live in poverty?
How does it feel to know that Black and Brown boys get expelled faster than any other race?
How does it feel to scream at the top of your lungs and no one hears you?
How does it feel to be a problem?

A problem is often seen as something negative, unwelcomed, harmful and needing to be "dealt with"
A problem can also be defined as an unexpected disruption in a system
So, my answer to the question, "How does it feel to be a problem?"
IS THAT YOU WERE BORN TO BE A PROBLEM!

You were not created to just go along to get along
The blood that flows through your veins is the same blood that beat through the hearts of men and women that were a problem
People that were born to disrupt the system, that challenged the status quo
People that dared to believe that this world could be different

Toussaint Louverture was a problem
Frederick Douglass was a problem
Harriet Tubman was a problem
Nat Turner was a problem
Jackie Robinson was a problem
Fannie Lou Hamer was a problem
Martin Luther King was a problem
Marcus Garvey was a problem
Fred Hampton was a problem
Malcom X was a problem
Assata Shakur was a problem
Barack Obama was a problem
Trayvon Martin, Sandra Bland and Mike Brown was a problem that shook a sleeping nation to a movement
You were born to be a problem!

You were created to disrupt the system
You are here to challenge the status quo
You are designed to question those in authority, to ask the hard questions

Why are you afraid of my Blackness?

Why is my wallet always seen as a gun?

Why is it okay to take healthcare away from those that might need it the most?

Why are we abusing people that want to protect the right to have clean water?

Why do women still get paid less than men for doing the same job?

Why do 62 people Hold As Much Wealth As The Poorest 3.5 Billion in the world?

Why does my zip code determine my life expectancy?

Why do you incarcerate more Black and Brown males than any other race?

Why does the educational system expel us at an alarming rate?

Why is the drug epidemic now a health crisis when years ago, no one cared when crack was ravishing the Black community?

Why can't I shop or eat a balanced meal in my own neighborhood?

Why do you turn your backs on the very people whose backs you walked on to build a nation?

Why does my existence threaten you?

Your job is to ask why?!

You were born to be a problem!

Because you were born with possibility, power, promise and potential

You were created to confront injustice

To be a thorn in the side of inequality!

You were made to be a voice for the voiceless

You see, you be that glitch in the Matrix!

If you were not a problem

They wouldn't be after you so hard

If you were not a problem

They wouldn't create laws to hold you back

If you were not a problem

They wouldn't try to squash your dreams

If you were not a problem

They wouldn't try to beat you down!

If you were not a problem

They wouldn't care about you organizing

If you were not a problem

They wouldn't infiltrate your community with drugs and alcohol

If you were not a problem

They wouldn't care that you stand up in your community

The reason they are after you is because they see your power

Because Strength always overpowers weakness

Light always outshines darkness

Like Thomas Merton said,

"How do I begin to tell you that you are all walking around shining like the sun?"

So, when they ask you, "How does it feel to be a problem?"

Stand proud, stand strong, stand in your authority and declare,

"IT FEELS AMAZING BECAUSE I WAS BORN TO BE A PROBLEM!"

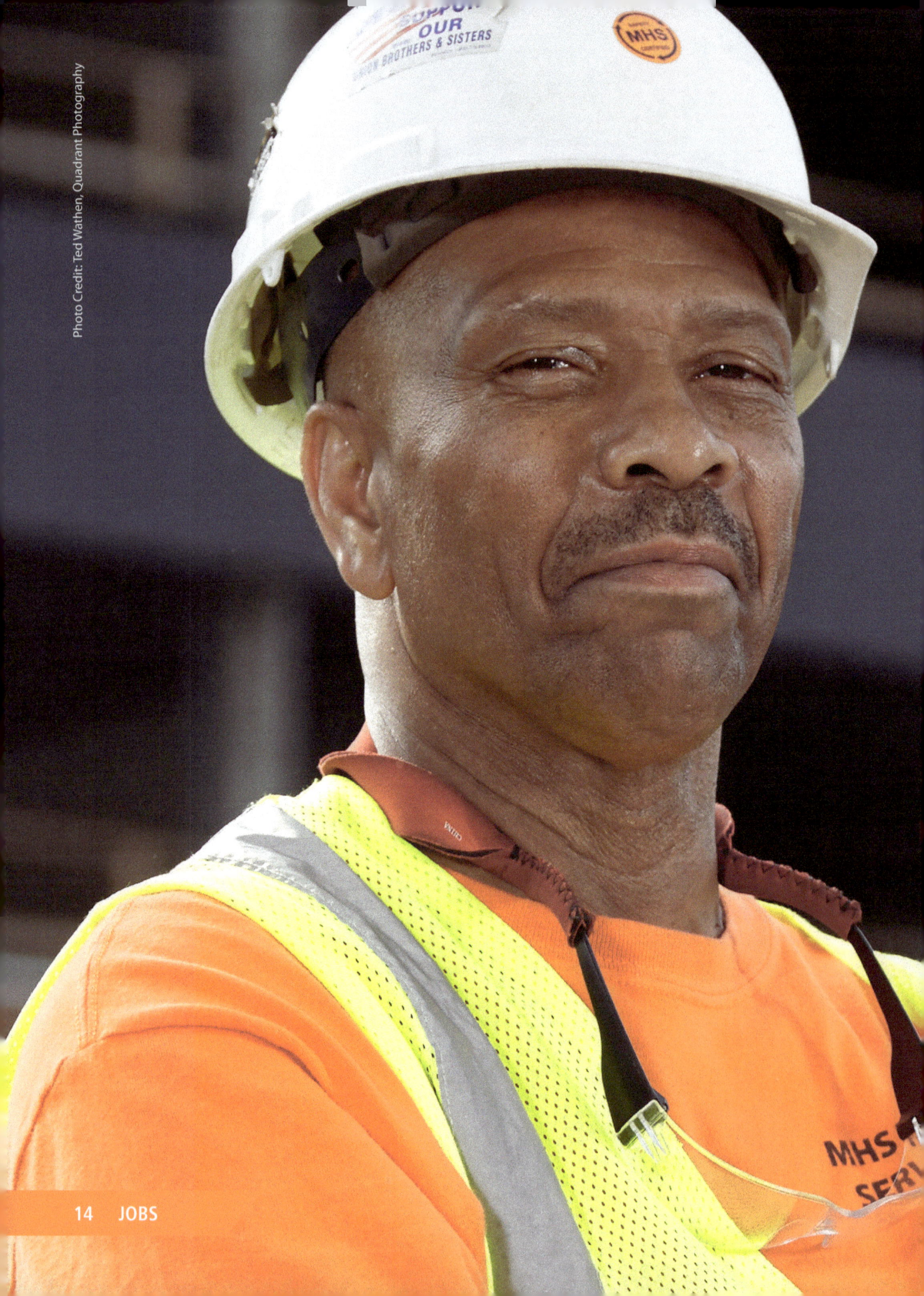

JOBS
AND ECONOMIC OPPORTUNITIES

Issues of poverty are directly related to justice, education, health, and housing. In Louisville, 15% of Whites live in poverty compared to 35.4% of African Americans.[4]

We must work to ensure that every resident has an equal opportunity to achieve economic success, sustainability, and financial security. In 2016, the Black unemployment rate in Louisville was more than double that of White residents: about 11% versus 5%.[5] Both the public and private sectors should support job-training programs and other efforts by the Louisville Urban League to address issues related to unemployment and under-employment. They should work to ensure that these programs are fully funded, supported, and expanded.

Our state government should do a better job in setting examples for local governments to follow. Among many other areas related to jobs and economic justice, we must call on local and state economic development councils, chambers of commerce, and the like to join with the Urban League and other community-based groups to study and develop concrete plans of action that address:

▶ Ensuring that African Americans have an equal opportunity to develop and to expand business opportunities;

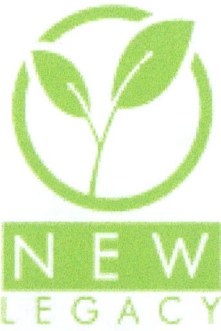

GISELA NELSON, New Legacy Reentry Corporation

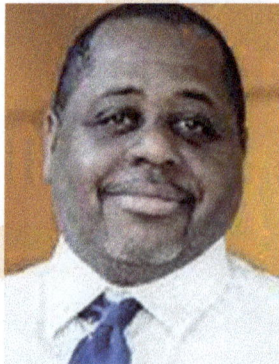

BILL HUSTON, New Legacy Reentry Corporation

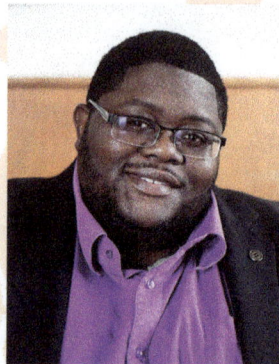

TED GATLIN, JR., Louisville Urban League Young Professionals

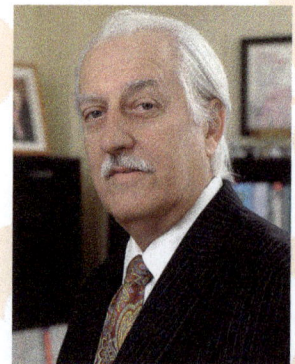

DR. CRAIG BLAKELY, University of Louisville

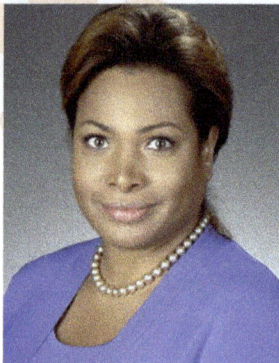

DR. KAREN CHAVIS, University of Louisville

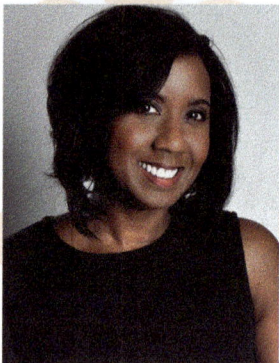

NIKKI R. JACKSON, Louisville Branch of the Federal Reserve Bank of St. Louis

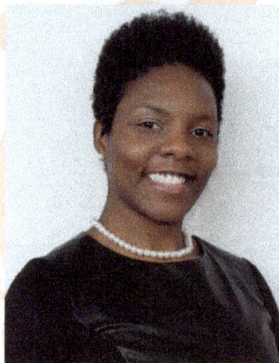

SHANDELIER BOYD SMITH, Louisville Urban League

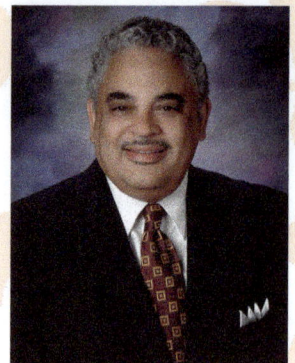

JOHN J. JOHNSON, Kentucky Commission on Human Rights

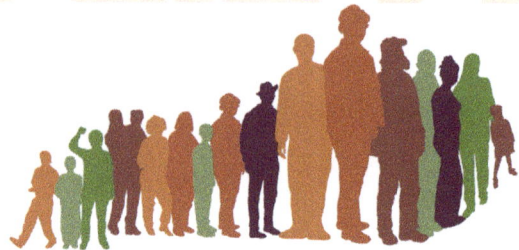

KENTUCKIANS FOR THE COMMONWEALTH

ECONOMIC JUSTICE COMMITTEE, Kentuckians For The Commonwealth

▶ Contracting and vendor supply opportunities must be enhanced for minority vendors;

▶ Assuring that minority businesses are able to compete for contract opportunities through the ability to secure bonding and adequate lines of credit.

Among other issues related to economic justice, we must address the predatory practices of payday lending and check cashing businesses in our communities.

John J. Johnson, Executive Director
Kentucky Commission on Human Rights

REDIRECTING THE NARRATIVE THROUGH COMMUNITY-BASED REENTRY

Gisela Nelson, Executive Director
Bill Huston, Business Development Director
New Legacy Reentry Corporation

Few criminal justice issues are more troubling than the prevalence of mass incarceration and the racial disparity within the criminal justice system – at all stages of the system beginning with arrest and proceeding through imprisonment, parole, and release. Substantial racial and ethnic disparities are found in virtually all jurisdictions in the United States, but we will drill down on Jefferson County, Kentucky.

We must understand the broader implications of mass incarceration and its impact on Black males in our community. Mass incarceration is correctional control; many Black males who are not physically incarcerated are being monitored daily by probation officers and parole officers and, thereby, subject to stop, search, and seizure without any probable cause or reasonable suspicion.

The criminal justice system is a massive apparatus, a system of direct control, and of course this doesn't even speak to the number of Black males who now have criminal records that are subject to legalized discrimination for the rest of their lives. These racial disparities have persisted for years. In many respects they have been exacerbated in recent years despite considerable social and economic progress in many areas of American life. Racist statutes within the legal code have been in existence in this country since its earliest foundation.

For many Black males who enter the criminal justice system, discriminatory sentencing patterns are often an unavoidable reality. Black men bear the brunt of the direct effects of serving time behind bars, with the effects lasting long after they leave prison and parole. Yet, the larger spillover effects are also extraordinarily racially unequal for Black and White families and communities.

Connections to family members in prison range from 6% for White males to 44% for Black females. Black women are far more likely than White women to know people in prison: 35% versus 15% for personal acquaintances; 44% versus 12% for family members; 22% versus 4% for neighbors; 17% versus 5% for someone they trust. Remarkably, the proportion of incarcerated individuals in the family network of an average Black female is 8.5 times higher than for the typical White woman.[6]

Louisville Metro is the largest city in Kentucky. Louisville is 21.56% Black with a 2017 Black population of 165,861[7] and half of that population is concentrated in five zip codes with populations over 55% Black (40202, 40203, 40210, 40211, and 40212)[8]. Louisville contains 49.1% of Kentucky's Black population[9]. Blacks in Louisville were 2.6 times more likely to be arrested by Louisville Metro Police than Whites. In fact, Blacks were 6.6 times more likely to be arrested by St. Matthews Police, the highest ratio in the state.[10] Black people represented 43.7% of the 62,532 arrests reported to the FBI by Metro Police in 2012, the most recent data studied. These disparities make reentry and recidivism paramount issues that must be addressed in Louisville's Black community.

The current general perception is that when someone is released from a period of incarceration, they should return to the same economic, educational, and racial disparities that spawned them and then they are expected to "make a life". This would all make sense if while incarcerated inmates were provided a continuum of rehabilitation services, but how can you *rehabilitate* someone who has not been *habilitated*?

The reality is that most Black male ex-offenders are "coming to five Louisville zip codes near you" and as a community it is all of our duty to assist in the reentry of returning citizens. We must work with community partners, employers, education providers, and state agencies to increase community safety, dispel prejudice and judgement, and reduce recidivism rates. There is a need for culturally-specific reentry programs to engage young Black males – from juveniles to young adults. These programs must engage the entire person and prepare them to reenter our Louisville communities and create businesses and jobs in their communities through

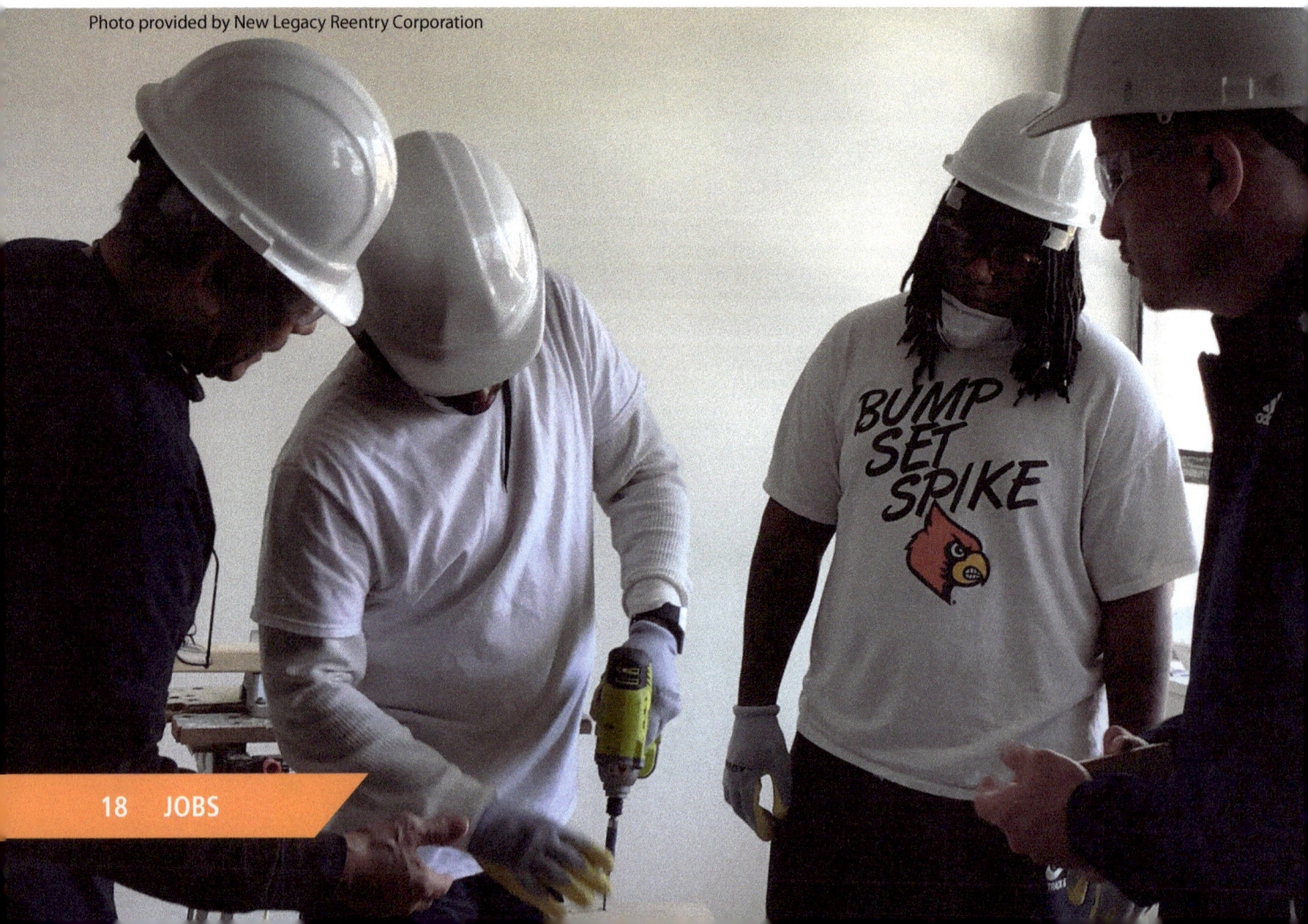

Photo provided by New Legacy Reentry Corporation

entrepreneurship and relevant job training programs.

HEAT Time is a comprehensive, uniquely-innovative, social justice consulting firm that addresses the most pressing reentry issues that impact our communities. HEAT Time applies holistic, culturally-relevant, responsive, strength-based models that emphasize positive and engaging approaches to healing individuals, families, and communities.

There is also a high concentration of returning citizens who come home to impoverished communities ill-equipped to provide the resources and services they and their families may need to smoothly transition into society. The largest hurdle for most returning citizens is securing gainful employment with a living wage. Legal and practical barriers often prevent them from accessing employment to earn a living wage and move out of or avoid poverty.

Entrepreneurship has emerged as a viable alternative to traditional employment opportunities for disadvantaged and marginalized individuals. The microenterprise development field, in particular, has demonstrated success assisting the hard-to-employ people and help them transcend poverty through business startup and development. New Legacy partners with other community organizations to create micro-enterprise opportunities for returning citizens while providing holistic programming to reduce recidivism.

Lastly, Kentucky excludes 26% of its Black population from the electoral process due to felony convictions.[11] That's nearly 70,000 people, and half of that population lives in those five concentrated zip codes in Metro Louisville. Restoration of civil rights is another vital area where the reentry community must make inroads to fully integrate our returning citizens to full citizenship and democratic participation. The signing of House Bill 40 on July 15th, 2016 allows Kentuckians convicted of certain Class D felonies to apply for expungement five years after they complete

their jail time, parole or probation. In Kentucky, a felony is a crime that is punishable by one year or more in state prison, with a Class D felony being punishable by one to five years. Convictions can be expunged through an application process. If the court grants the application, the original judgment will be vacated and the charges dismissed. Records in the custody of any other agency or official, including law enforcement records, will be expunged.

Expungement reform will help employers find qualified employees to fill vacant positions and allow tens of thousands of Kentuckians to better support themselves and their families.

TO BE YOUNG, PROFESSIONAL, AND BLACK… IN LOUISVILLE

Ted Gatlin, Jr., Founder; President
Unlimited Results Experiential Training and Development
Louisville Urban League Young Professionals

Louisville is a place with an identity crisis. It›s fighting to be a small town while at the same time trying to be an international-level city. This means there is still a good old boy network at play in most arenas while a facade of professional opportunities exist for certain people of color, just enough to register on the "we are not a racist community scale."

This identity crisis affects the young, Black, professional community in very specific ways, both professionally and socially. It creates professional blockades and cliques that depress the energy of the young, Black professional and, in the end, contributes to a drain of talent.

I have been part of the Louisville Urban League Young Professionals since 2011. I currently serve as president. In this position, I have found myself in boardrooms that I would not have been invited into in any other case. What I have found most interesting as I have navigated is the lack of other people of color in these same spaces. I can usually find Black professionals in entry-level and lower-level management roles. I typically can also find at least one exceptional senior-level person of color, but in those decision-making roles, those people on the rise, those on the cusp of real leadership, we are noticeably absent. The real question is why? I believe the answer is: Louisville does not care about the young, Black professional.

It shows up in many ways. You see it in the lack of opportunities given for personal and professional development at many of the top companies. You see it with the pressure applied to be the best, stay the latest, and overachieve just to be considered good enough to handle low-level management. You see it when corporations are asked for their best and brightest, and a call goes out for the ones that same network already knows.

I understand that it's also incumbent upon the young,

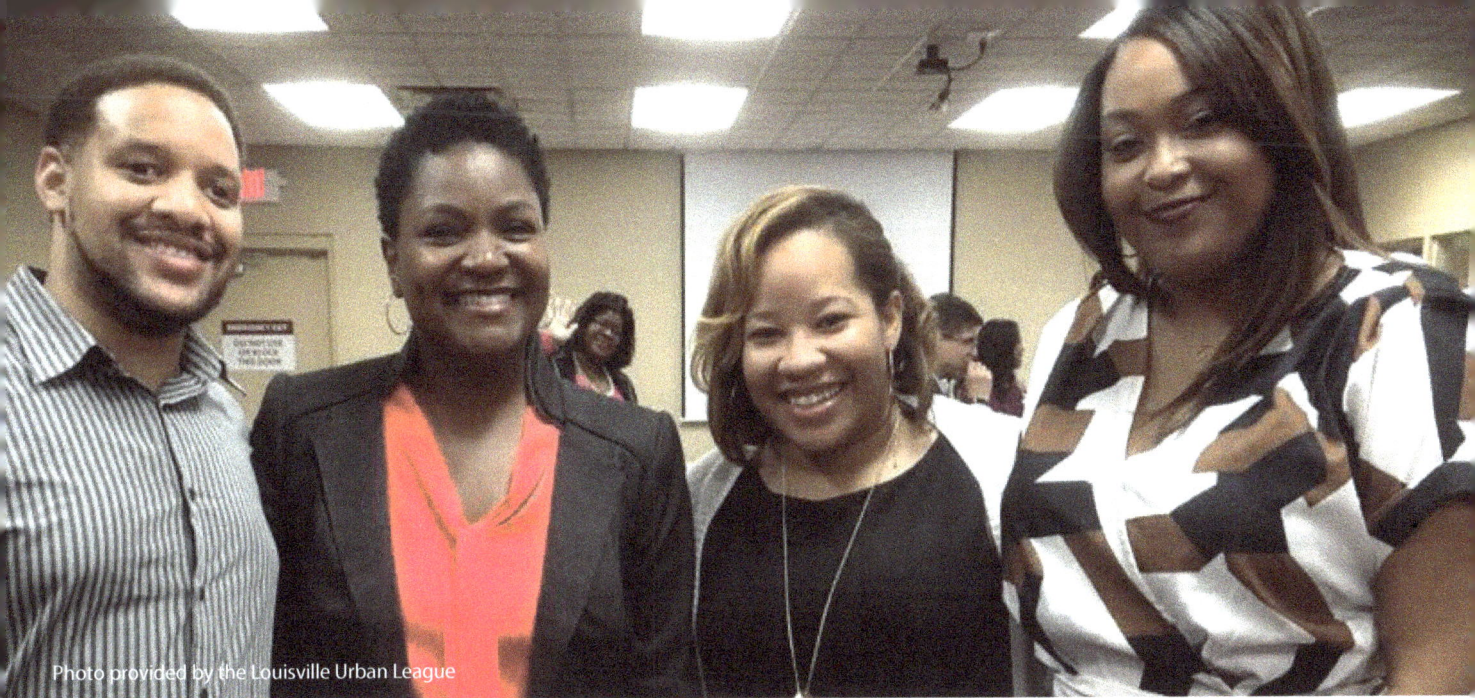

Photo provided by the Louisville Urban League

Black professional to network and get themselves in a position to be seen. Although this is true, in reality, those who do break through often end up in a situation where they are not able or, in some cases, willing to build a bridge for other young, Black professionals. They become part of the good old boy network instead of transforming the network that continues the cycle of exclusivity at true leadership levels.

Socially, Louisville has potential for the young, Black professional. There is a need for Black professionals to congregate with one another socially; however, diverse opportunities are few and far between. Often, activities are similar in design or contain the same people. Additionally, finding the group you best "fit" with can be daunting, especially if you are a transplant or a person who isn't one to go out and socialize. There is a definite need for more "for us, by us" type of events, but there is also a need for young, Black professionals to put in the work to attend and participate. In wondering why there seems to be a dearth of diversity in attendees, most young, Black professionals cite work as the overriding factor.

This brings me to an epiphany. Young, Black professionals end up putting in so much work at their jobs to be seen and to be excellent in order to move

up, that social interactions become less important or become just a function of their job. The dull, after-work scene is likely an effect of the emotional labor exhibited during the 9-5.

So what's the fix? Louisville's Black professionals need to put a priority on congregating with one another while participating in diverse events and spaces. We need to get out of the mindset of wondering who is going to be there, and just take ourselves there. Louisville corporations need to immediately – in unapologetic terms – promote young, Black professionals for opportunities to gain development. Corporations need to support their professionals' outside activities within the community that help them to become a more rounded employee. Black professionals in upper leadership need to be always looking for a young professional to mentor, as this is the only way to actively infiltrate the good old boy network that persists.

BLACK EMPLOYMENT AT LOUISVILLE'S PREMIER RESEARCH INSTITUTION: ONE INTROSPECTIVE REFLECTION

Dr. Craig Blakely, Dean
School of Public Health and Information Sciences, University of Louisville

Dr. Karan Chavis, Chief of Staff
School of Medicine, University of Louisville

Perhaps the single most important demographic at the University of Louisville, with respect to diversity, is the proportion of Black students on campus – 10.2% in the fall 2016. However, for the purposes of this exploration of Black in Louisville, we are more directly concerned about employment at the university as indicated by the proportions of Blacks within key university employment categories. By way of context, the state population is less than 10% Black, while the Louisville metro area is roughly one quarter Black.[12]

Like most major employers in the city, the university's strategic efforts point toward ensuring equal access to employment and a workplace free of barriers and harassment. Every job search document includes the boilerplate language committing the institution to being an equal opportunity affirmative action employer. Examining diversity in the workplace at the university, we quickly find evidence of success in the institutional metrics that reflect those strategic plans.

The data behind the university's 2016 Affirmative Action Plan provide a picture of the employment patterns of the university. At the executive level, in 2015, Blacks filled 8.5% of the key positions in the President's Office and the Office of the Provost. In the faculty ranks, 5.5% were Black.[13] This central figure is a bit disappointing. In some cases, the profession is not diverse, thus it is extremely difficult to make Black hires in that academic arena. Nevertheless, despite evidence of progress, more can be done.

In the ranks of professionals – those non-faculty hires such as counselors, librarians, purchasing experts, finance staff, academic advisors, – Blacks accounted for 9.3% of those on payroll. In office support roles, the proportion increases to 14.6%. In the technical professional category – electrical science technicians, printing technicians, lab technicians – Blacks filled 10.1% of the slots. In skilled trades, Blacks filled 8.3% of the jobs. In the service/maintenance, Blacks filled 52.7% of the positions. Examining these

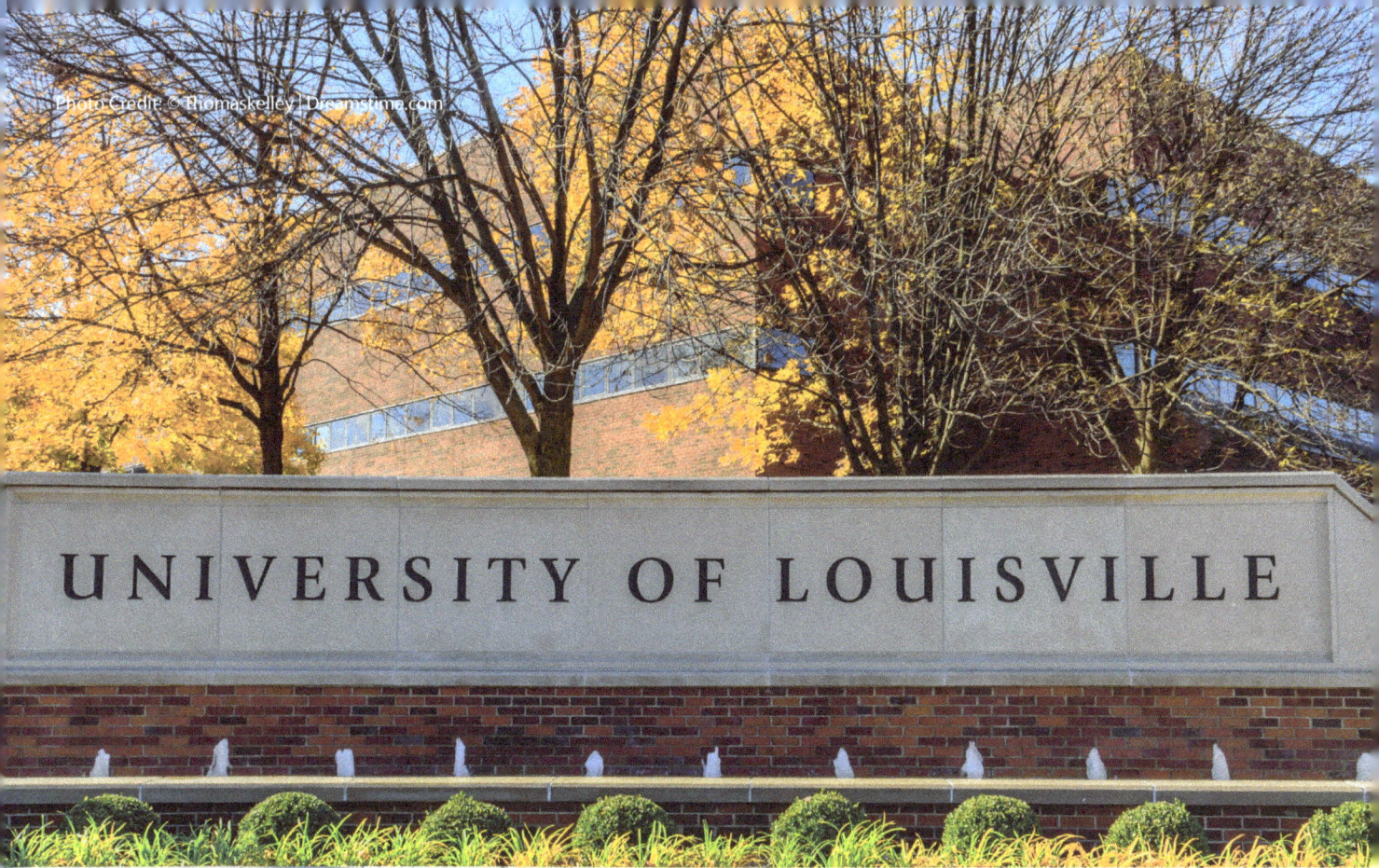

figures by category begs the question whether grounds maintenance and janitorial jobs are the primary opportunities for Black employment at the university. Further, are opportunities less available for employment in more skilled trades or supervisory roles?

Perhaps these data reflect a failed process of monitoring of the metrics and responding, rather than a true institutional barrier to equal access to advancement. However, that question is far less important than what the university chooses to do with these data now that they have been dissected and displayed so succinctly. Our institutions must make contributions, top to bottom, if we are to participate in the creation of a climate in Louisville that allows Black residents to meaningfully expect to access a reasonable slice of the American Dream. We need considerably more help from Washington D.C., and Frankfort to pull this off, but we have no right to expect that help if we continue to fail to identify our local shortcomings and bring about change right

here at home.

We must and do recognize our shortcomings and are committed to quality improvement efforts. We hope that the other major employers in our community also overtly explore their metrics on diversity at all levels of the workforce, for only together can we begin to change the climate in Louisville and, in particular, west Louisville where an average of 74.2% of the residents in its five primary zip codes are Black.[14] We know that improvements to the economic foundations of employees and their families extend to improvements in other aspects of quality of life indicators such as educational attainment of children, housing opportunities, and the social determinants of health. Together, can we create an environment where we all have reason to believe we can be successful.

THE RACIAL WEALTH GAP: ADDRESSING THE REASONS AND POSSIBLE SOLUTIONS

Nikki R. Jackson, Senior Vice President
Louisville Branch of the Federal Reserve Bank of St. Louis

The opinions expressed below are not attributable to the Federal Reserve System.

My colleagues at the Federal Reserve Bank of St. Louis' Center for Household Financial Stability have observed that Blacks with college degrees have lost wealth over the past generation.

Center research, led by William Emmons and Bryan Noeth, found that between 1992 and 2013, college-educated Whites saw their wealth soar by 86% while college-educated Blacks saw theirs plummet by 55%.[15] Both Black and White college graduates enjoyed wealth gains between 2013 and 2016, but the median Black college graduate's wealth in 2016 remained below its 1992 level.

Seeing these numbers gave me reason to pause and ask more questions. Was there an advantage that college-educated Whites had over college-educated Blacks? And if so, let's get to the bottom

Median Net-Worth Figures for College-Graduate Families

	BLACK	WHITE
1992	$76,142	$199,358
2013	$34,521	$371,820
2016	$65,821	$389,801

of the mystery. As Ray Boshara, the Center's director noted in a Washington Post op-ed published last April, "Losing wealth means losing a cushion against hard times and a springboard for better times; it also means losing a chance to endow the next generation with the wealth we've accumulated over our lives."[16]

The Center team further questioned how college-educated Blacks over the past 25 years actually lost wealth despite meaningful progress in educational attainment, political representation, voting rights, anti-discrimination measures, and other realms. To address this puzzle, the center organized a research symposium with leading scholars from around the U.S. Here are some of their findings, many of which Boshara summarized in the Washington Post op-ed.

One of the key findings was the racial differences around preparing for college and financing college. The research showed that Black college grads are more likely than White college grads to have needed more student loans. This of course would lead to a negative effect on wealth because student loans defer or displace wealth-building measures such as marriage, buying a home, and saving for retirement.

Other findings noted included homeownership, which is more common among college-educated families. It seems that, in comparison with all other races, Black college grads fell behind. Black mortgage borrowers – even before the financial crisis and well before any other racial and ethnic group – are far more likely than their White peers to

experience foreclosures and delinquencies. Seeing this report shows that there is work to be done and that there are long-term damaging effects to Black homeownership wealth.

While on the subject of home ownership, let's look at some other statistics reported in 2015 by Louisville's Metropolitan Housing Coalition.[17] They found that in Jefferson County, 71% of White households are owner-occupied, compared with 37.5% of Black households. Of the 63% of all owner-occupied households, only 12% were Black. It appears the Louisville homeownership rate is a bit above the national average, but I have not seen any data to suggest the low ownership trend for Black families is different than the national average. It is without dispute, however, that homeownership is a major factor in the level and volatility of overall wealth, especially for African American and Latino families.

Third, as stated in the op-ed, Black and White graduates share and receive wealth among their families quite differently. The key component seems

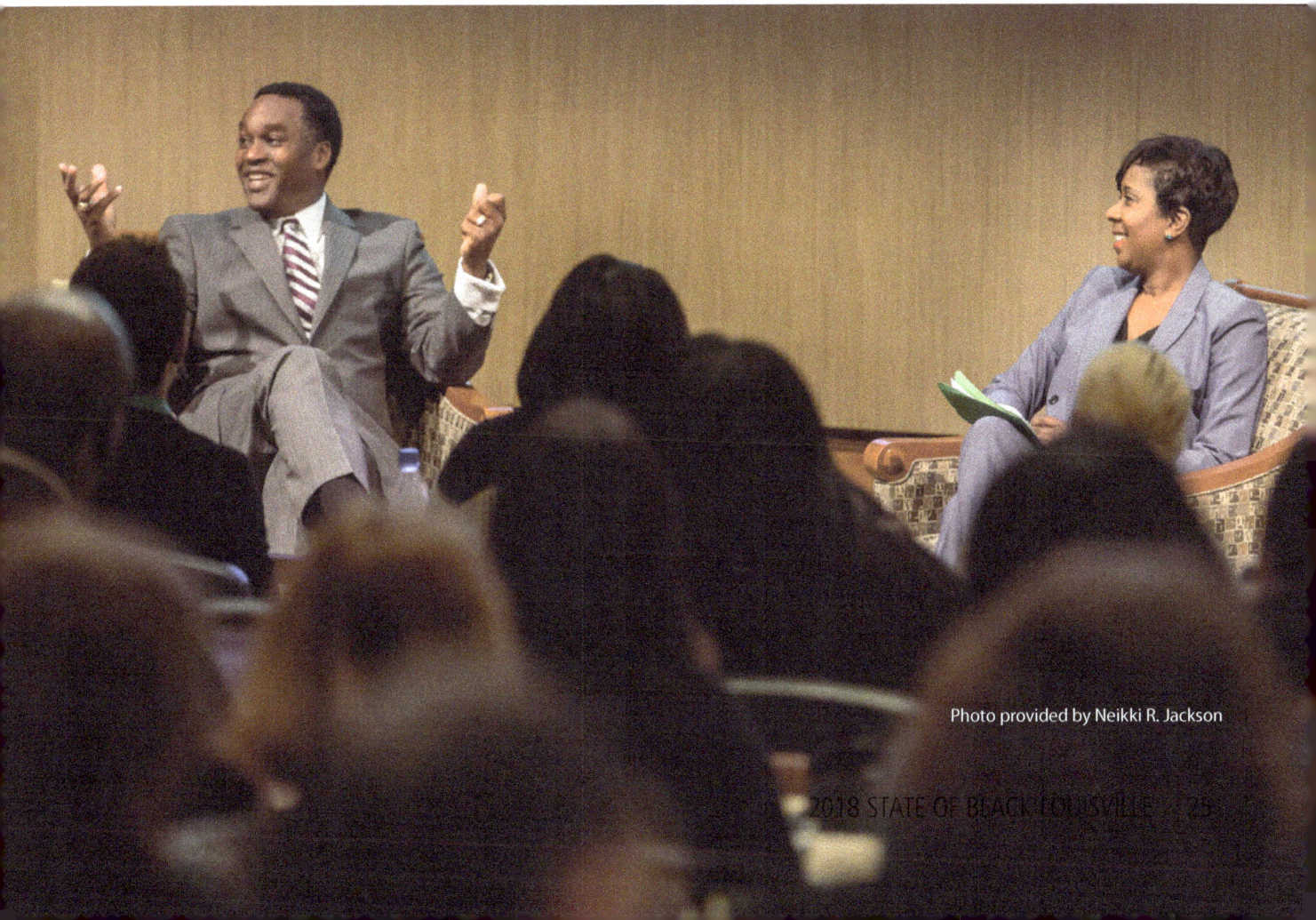

Photo provided by Neikki R. Jackson

to be the financial assistance White students get as a whole compared to Black students. College-educated Whites are more likely than college-educated Blacks to receive various levels of financial assistance from parents. Not only do college-educated Blacks not receive as much financial assistance, if any, they are more likely to end up in a situation where they are providing financial assistance to their struggling parents or extended family in need. These financial hardships play out for college-educated Blacks despite their lower incomes and wealth. It should be noted that wealth-sharing includes transfers at the end of life as well as throughout, such as for private K-12 schooling, college, a first home, or averting a cash-flow crisis, to name a few.

Finally, as we look again at what was stated in the op-ed and the findings from Emmons and Center Lead Analyst Lowell Ricketts in their symposium paper, it seems we can't ignore these historical experiences and ongoing discrimination. Nor, after looking at all that has been presented to us, can we fault Blacks by claiming that they just made poor decisions. The standard but debatable "post-racial" economic model, under which the racial wealth gap exists because millions of White families made good financial choices while millions of similarly-situated Black families did not, is disrupted by Emmons and Ricketts' model because the Black-White wealth gap is too large and persistent for equal opportunity and freedom of choice to be plausible.

So how do we address racism's role in wealth attainment? How do we work together to build a more equitable society that focuses on all affected, and not just an individual? These symposium findings have shown us that policies, along with bold programs, are required to reset the racial wealth gaps in America. Some of the solutions discussed with my colleagues include tackling the attainment of college degrees, diversified savings, and debt reduction. We might also look at some of the following suggestions, as outlined in the Washington Post op-ed:

- ▶ Financing higher education with less debt and more grants, scholarships, and savings could help, as could homeownership reforms that build economic resilience through more equity financing, savings, and insurance.

- ▶ For families without access to financial assistance from extended family, pools of financial capital (from lending circles and matched savings programs, for example) could be expanded to propel upward economic mobility.

- ▶ A bold program of "baby bonds," or wealth endowments at birth for lower-wealth households that are earmarked for lifelong asset accumulation, could be launched.

It's difficult to talk about the impact of current day structural and institutional racism without also acknowledging its roots: slavery, Jim Crow, and the state of civil and voting rights for African Americans and Latinos. To the extent those conversations are shunned or muted by those in positions to dismantle those pervasive structures and institutions, we are less likely to make real progress on this critical issue.

BUDGETS ARE MORAL DOCUMENTS: KENTUCKY'S GENERAL FUND AND PROGRESSIVE TAX REFORM

Economic Justice Committee
Kentuckians For The Commonwealth

A budget reflects a community's values and vision. It's how we pool resources, accomplishing together what we can't accomplish alone. Kentucky's state budget should reflect needs and priorities that lead toward a just, equitable, and vibrant commonwealth.

KENTUCKY'S GENERAL FUND

The Kentucky General Fund budget is about $20.3 billion dollars over a two-year term.[18] It funds:

▶ Education, including early childhood education, K-12, higher education, need-based scholarships, and arts and heritage programs

▶ Health care, including care for low-income folks, people with disabilities, elderly Kentuckians, and public health services

▶ Human services and supports, including child and domestic violence prevention, foster care and adoption services, and Medicaid waivers

▶ Infrastructure, including roads, public transit, and water and sewer systems

▶ Environmental protection, including land use, environmental safeguards for clean water and air, state parks, and home weatherization services

▶ Public safety and justice, including disaster relief and public defense

▶ Economic and workforce development, including workforce training, tourism, and small business development

Kentucky's General Fund is funded largely by tax dollars. Individual income taxes, sales taxes, corporate income taxes, and property taxes are the largest buckets of revenue. There are also smaller sources of revenue such as cigarette tax, lottery revenue, and tobacco settlement funds. There's still a smaller category of tax revenue that includes the inheritance

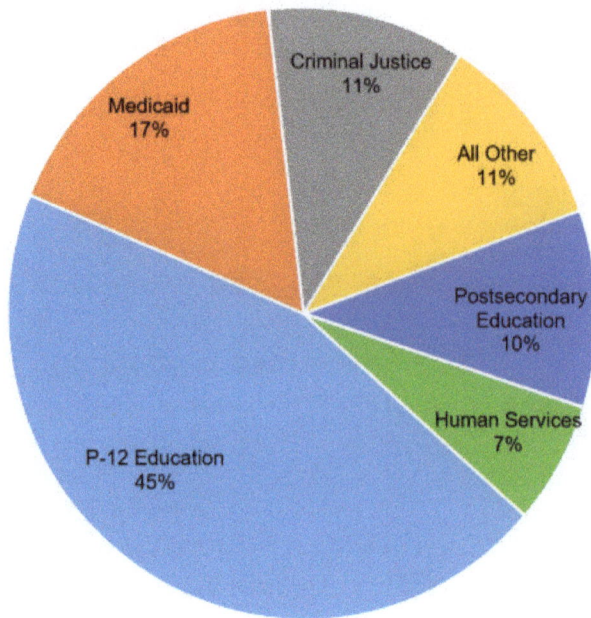

Figure 1: How General Fund Dollars are Spent[25]

tax, beer tax, bank franchise tax, etc., making up about 7% of General Fund revenue. Finally, in recent years, Fund Transfers have become a way to fund Kentucky's General Fund, with the legislature drawing from fees that are collected for the public worker health trust fund and criminal justice training. Kentucky also has a Rainy Day Fund, which could be used to supplement our General Fund in an emergency.

THE CURRENT CHALLENGES

Kentucky's public services and programs should work to give every Kentuckian the opportunity to succeed. Yet, we face a challenging moment. We have a state budget that is leaving us with less to invest, when we should be investing more for our future. Most of our state agencies have endured budget cuts of about 40% since 2008. These include the Kentucky Arts Council (-42%), Kentucky Educational Television (-32%), libraries (-26%), public health departments (-16%), the community college system (-27%), and vocational rehabilitation (-22%).[19]

After years of legislatures and governors not making the required contributions to our state pension funds, despite requiring employees to make and

increase their payments, our pension systems are at dangerously low funding levels. The Kentucky Budget Office's website shows the budget outlook would be tight even without big additional outlays for pensions.

Black communities in Louisville are among the communities that are disproportionately impacted by this crisis. Over the years, the inadequate tax revenue has led to an erosion of social services that support economic equity. Right now, it's not an equal playing field. Institutional racism has meant that Black communities in Louisville are deeply impacted by lower property values, a wealth gap, and an income gap. According to a report from the Kentucky Center for Economic Policy, the poverty rate in Kentucky between 2010 and 2012 was 17% for Whites and 34% for African Americans.[20] While more than half of working families of color in Kentucky are low income – a household income below $32,040 for a family of three – less than a third of White working families statewide are low income.[21]

Economic inequality, institutional racism, and gaps in opportunity that include an inequitable education system perpetuate poverty and low wages in Louisville's Black communities. These communities are also affected by the failure to invest in eroding public infrastructure, by unenforced environmental safeguards, by inequities in the justice system, a need for restorative justice, and food injustice.

Because Kentucky isn't addressing statewide funding challenges, Black communities in Louisville have been heavily impacted. Many public services have been cut as a result of lack of revenue such as pools in urban areas and after-school programs for the youth. Louisville must patch together Band-Aids to deal with the disproportionate impact on lower-income residents. More money seems to go towards downtown development instead of into neighborhood development or affordable housing.

The impact of eroded public services ripples out

further. It increasingly marginalizes people, creates additional layers of distrust in public services, and casts doubt on the ability and willingness of our government to address the community's needs. This opens the door for further privatization of public services and even more so consolidates money and power to the already powerful.

POTENTIAL POLICY RECOMMENDATIONS

Recommended policies must be fair, especially to lower-income folks, and that should always be grounded in advancing equity. Comprehensive tax reform is a necessary next step to create a more equitable budget. These reforms must not disproportionately impact lower-income Kentuckians and communities that are already impacted by institutional racism.

The Kentucky Forward Plan, a comprehensive tax reform plan sponsored by Louisville's Representative Jim Wayne and supported by most of the Jefferson County Democratic Caucus, is the best example of tax reforms that would support a fairer, more equitable society.[22]

The Kentucky Forward Plan would:

▶ Create a 15% State Earned Income Tax Credit, which means that families who qualify for the federal EITC would qualify for an additional 15% from their Kentucky returns. A state EITC would offset chronically low wages, making it more feasible for low-income folks to hold a job.

▶ Modernize income tax brackets to make Kentucky's income tax more progressive, with higher tax rates on higher levels of income and by adding a tax bracket for millionaires. Currently in Kentucky, persons making over $150,000 dollars pay the top rate of 6% in state and local taxes. If, the state were to create a new tax bracket, persons making over $150,000 would now pay a top rate of 6.5 %.

▶ Close loopholes and handouts for corporations and developers. The state takes in about $10 billion, but gives out a little over $12 billion in tax breaks. Kentucky currently has 270 tax breaks on the book that need to be examined to see if they are helping or harming our economy.[23]

▶ Reduce the pension exclusion for wealthy retirees, eliminating the exclusion for retirement income over $70,000.

▶ Raise the cigarette tax to the national average. The national average is $1.60 per pack. Kentucky taxes cigarettes at 60 cents per pack. The Kentucky Chamber of Commerce supports an increase. Raising the cigarette tax also addresses a notorious public health issue: Kentucky has high rates for lung cancer and respiratory issues.[24]

Together, these policies would direct $115 million back into the pockets of working families, while raising about $580 million every year for Kentucky's public investments. These policies would be even more effective with an increase in Kentucky's minimum wage, and a more participatory democracy that would ensure that our budget reflects the values and priorities of all of us.

AN OPPORTUNITY TO RUN! HOW A TRACK CAN CHANGE EVERYTHING

Shandelier Boyd Smith, Kentucky Athletic Hall of Famer
Louisville Urban League

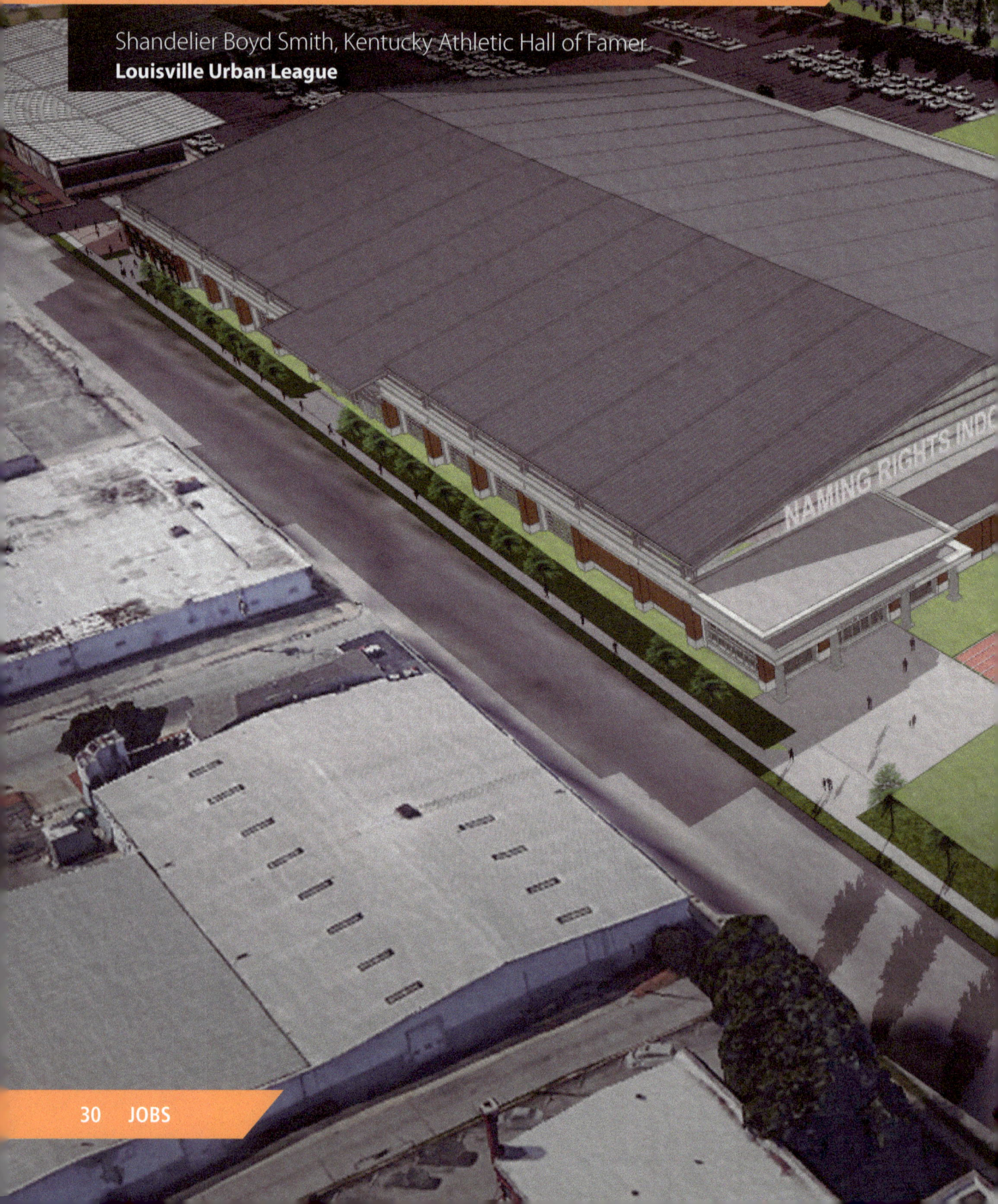

NAMING RIGHTS INDO

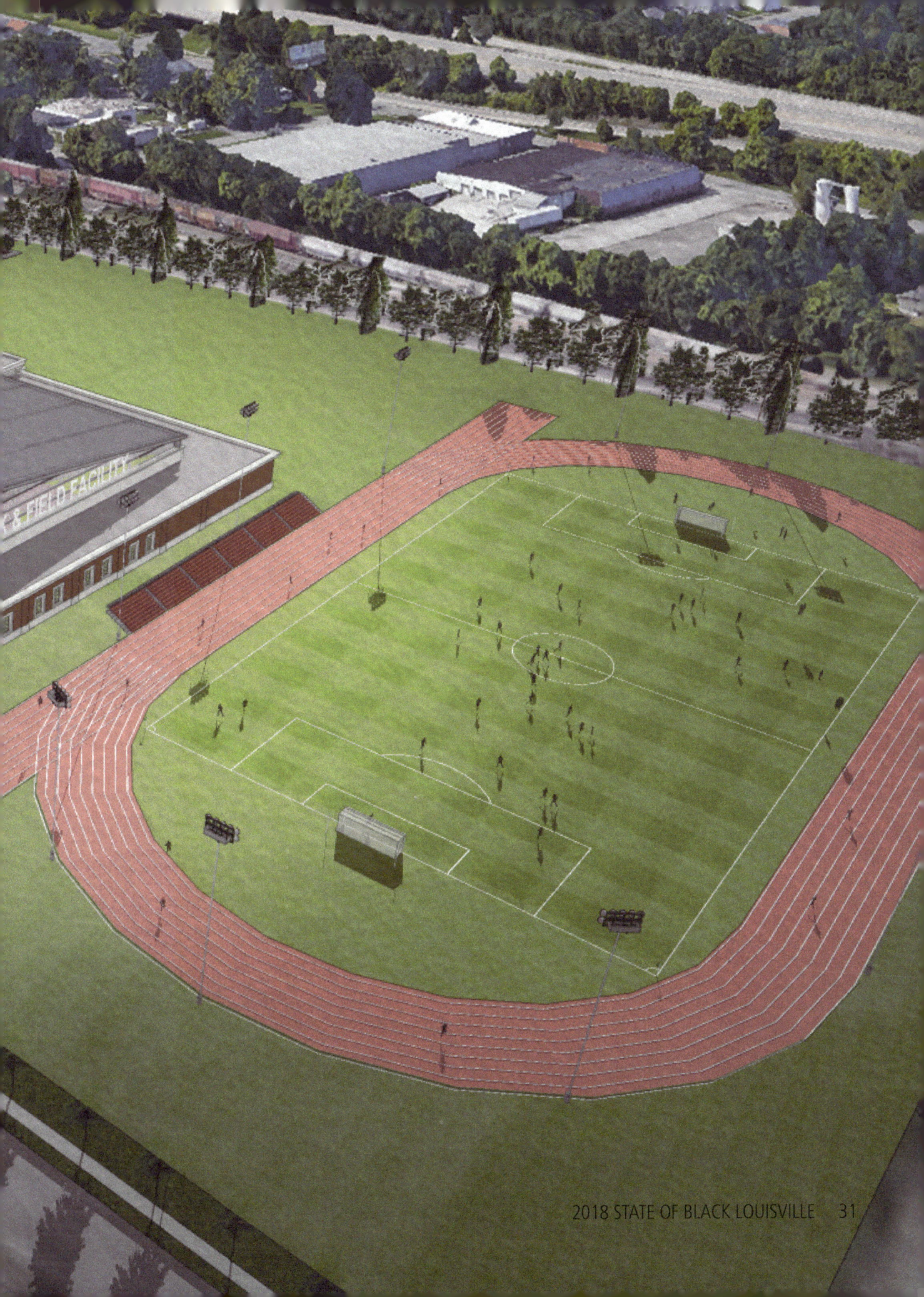

The city of Louisville and community leadership awarded the Louisville Urban League with the rights to develop and lead the effort to build a $30 million indoor track and field complex in the heart of west Louisville. It came after an extensive and competitive review process exploring the best use for the 24-acre campus located at 30th Street and West Muhammad Ali Boulevard in the Russell neighborhood. This is a project that will have lasting and sustainable impact on the economy, quality of life, health, and overall wellness of our entire community.

The plan for The Track on Ali is the result of a process driven by and including local residents. These are the voices with the highest investment and the biggest stake in the inequality crisis, and it's time that their voices are heard and action taken.

There have been a number of "plans" for west Louisville. Many of them have had some impact. Some of them have even had some lasting impact. Yet, none of them have held the promise that this project will provide. Our vision is to create a state-of-

the-art indoor track and field facility that is among the most admired in the country.

A LIFE-CHANGING EXPERIENCE

I'm from west Louisville and I'm still living by track.

As a child, I was very adventurous; a tomboy. I was always running and jumping and playing. I knew I was fast and everyone else knew it too, but we didn't know much about the sport of track. My mother used to exercise at Flaget Community Center. When I was about nine years old, she bumped into Kentucky High School Hall of Fame coach, William "Chico" Underwood, and asked him to give me a tryout. It stuck. I ran every summer with the Westside Track Club and that experience changed my life.

Track taught me perseverance. Coach Underwood would take me to train with older kids at local high schools where I was exposed to other people who were driven, disciplined, and willing to push their bodies to the limit to be the best at this sport. Track bolstered my self-confidence. Anytime I stepped

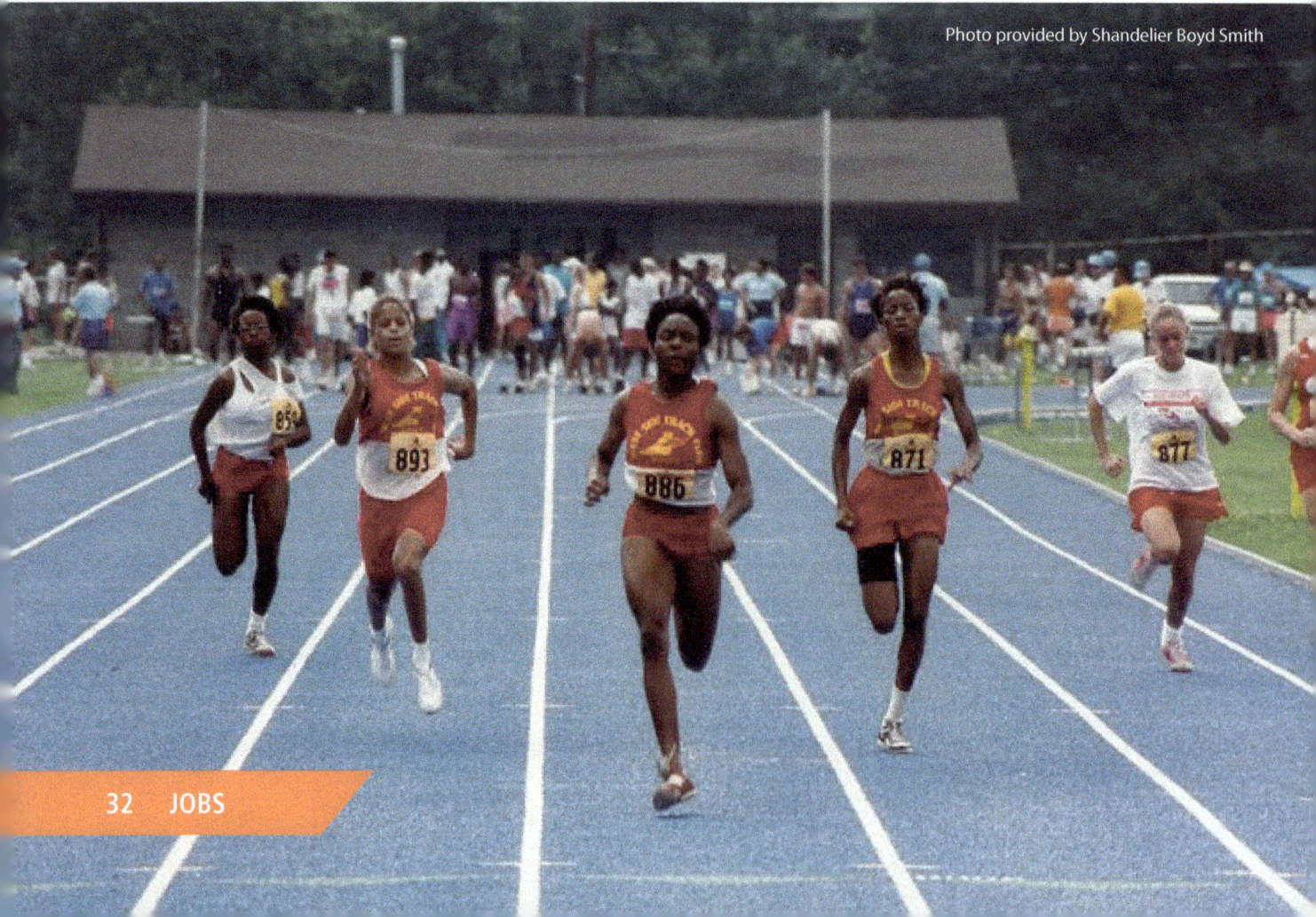

Photo provided by Shandelier Boyd Smith

to the line, I knew there was either a target on my back or, due to my size, a sea of doubters watching me. I learned how to manage that kind of pressure. Track allowed me to further my education. I attended a world-class university and earned a degree in a field I love. As I traveled, I experienced new cultures, learned new languages, and tried new foods. Beyond the degree track afforded me, I learned about the world.

Track taught me the importance of sacrifice. I didn't get to do a lot of the things others kids my age were doing at the time. Certainly, it kept me away from certain pitfalls like drugs or a premature pregnancy that snared some of my friends. But it also kept me from time with my friends, and trips to mall, and the other things teenagers do. But that sacrifice has afforded me the opportunity to meet remarkable people and see the world and be in spaces I could have never imagined.

At fourteen, I received an invite to the Hershey Invitational in Hershey, PA. It was my first time on an airplane and my first time to travel away by myself. As a high school freshman, I was able to compete and win at the Kentucky state championship. In the summer of 1992, I competed as a member of the U.S. Junior Olympic team in Seoul, South Korea – my first time out of the country. As a junior in college, I vividly remember lining up for the 60-meter hurdles against one of my heroes: gold medalist Jackie Joyner Kersey. I did not win.

Without even knowing it, track made me a leader in my own family. My parents introduced me to track and were my biggest supporters, ensuring that I always had everything I needed. They found a way to follow me all around the region to see me compete, even after my father lost his job. As my older brothers and sisters have cheered me on from trackside, they have also been inspired. Two of them returned to college to get their degrees, and the others have taken risks to move ahead in life. Risks, they say, were inspired by my success in sport and the classroom.

I have nieces and nephews who have gone on to college and been successful in sport and academia. Track has had an impact on generations.

SOMETHING TO ROOT FOR

In addition to being used by youth, high school, college, and university programs, The Track on Ali will attract regional runners and competition from across the country, including being able to host NCAA and USA Track and Field events. This is a change that will dramatically impact tourism in Louisville – increasing hotels stays and the utilization of local restaurants.

The Track on Ali will demolish barriers for families from outside of the community coming to west Louisville. Businesses, like healthy eateries and apparel stores, will grow out the need to serve top-tier athletes. Restaurants and boutique hotels could spring forth to serve families and fans. The phobias that many harbor about "this part of town" will be slowly chipped away as the track will be a magnet for west Louisville, creating new economic opportunities for all.

A state-of-the-art track facility will bring world-class athletes to the city. That exposure alone can change the world. I know, because it changed mine. My track experience showed me just how big the world is and how much more I had to learn. The Track on Ali will be an economic boon for west Louisville, and that is a wonderful thing. I can't help but be excited for the boys and girls whose lives will be forever changed by what they see, learn, and experience as they get a front row seat to watch and possibly compete in the sport I love. If my experience is any indicator, the Track on Ali represents an opportunity for kids, families, and communities to be positively and profoundly changed forever. How can anyone root against that?

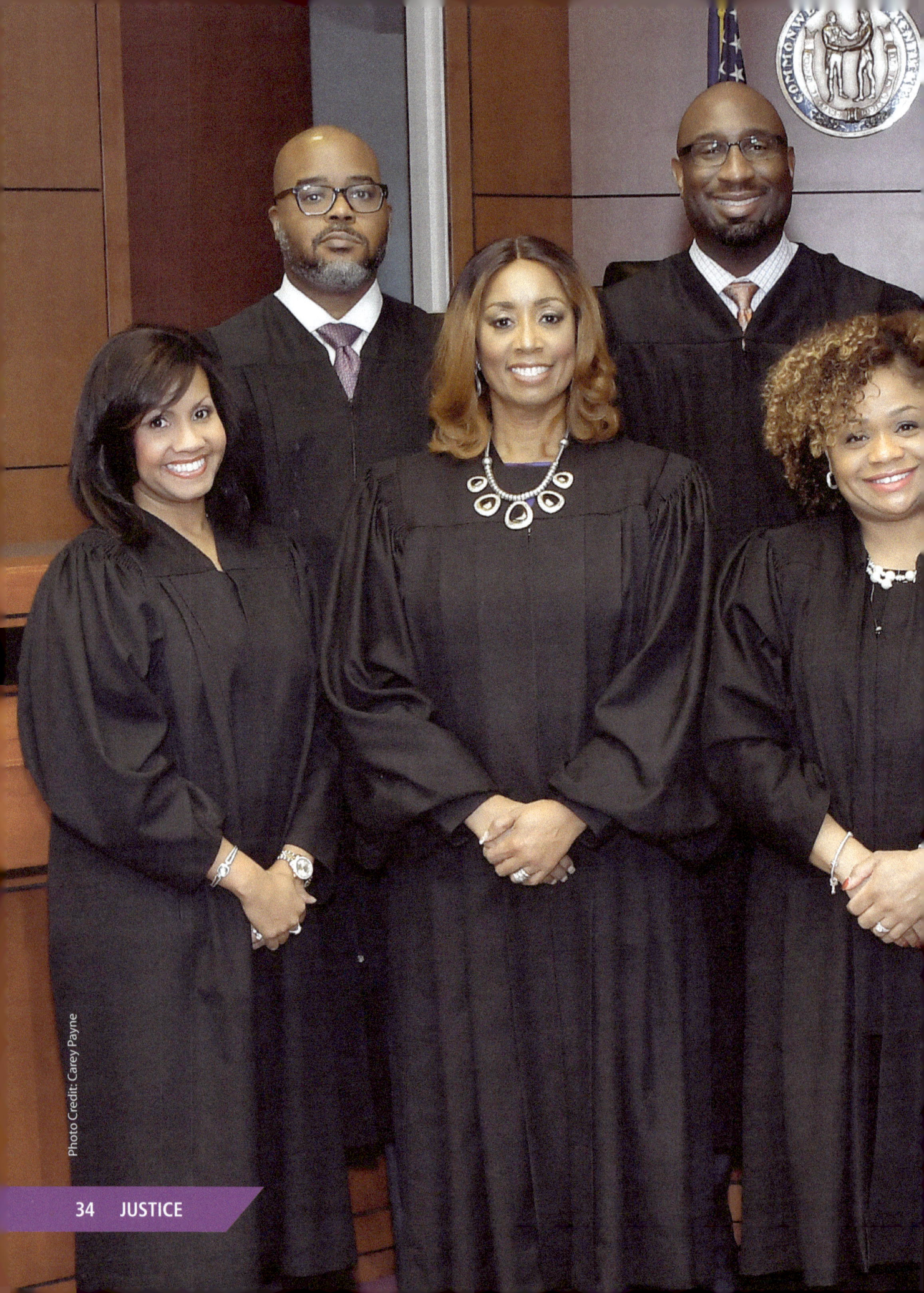

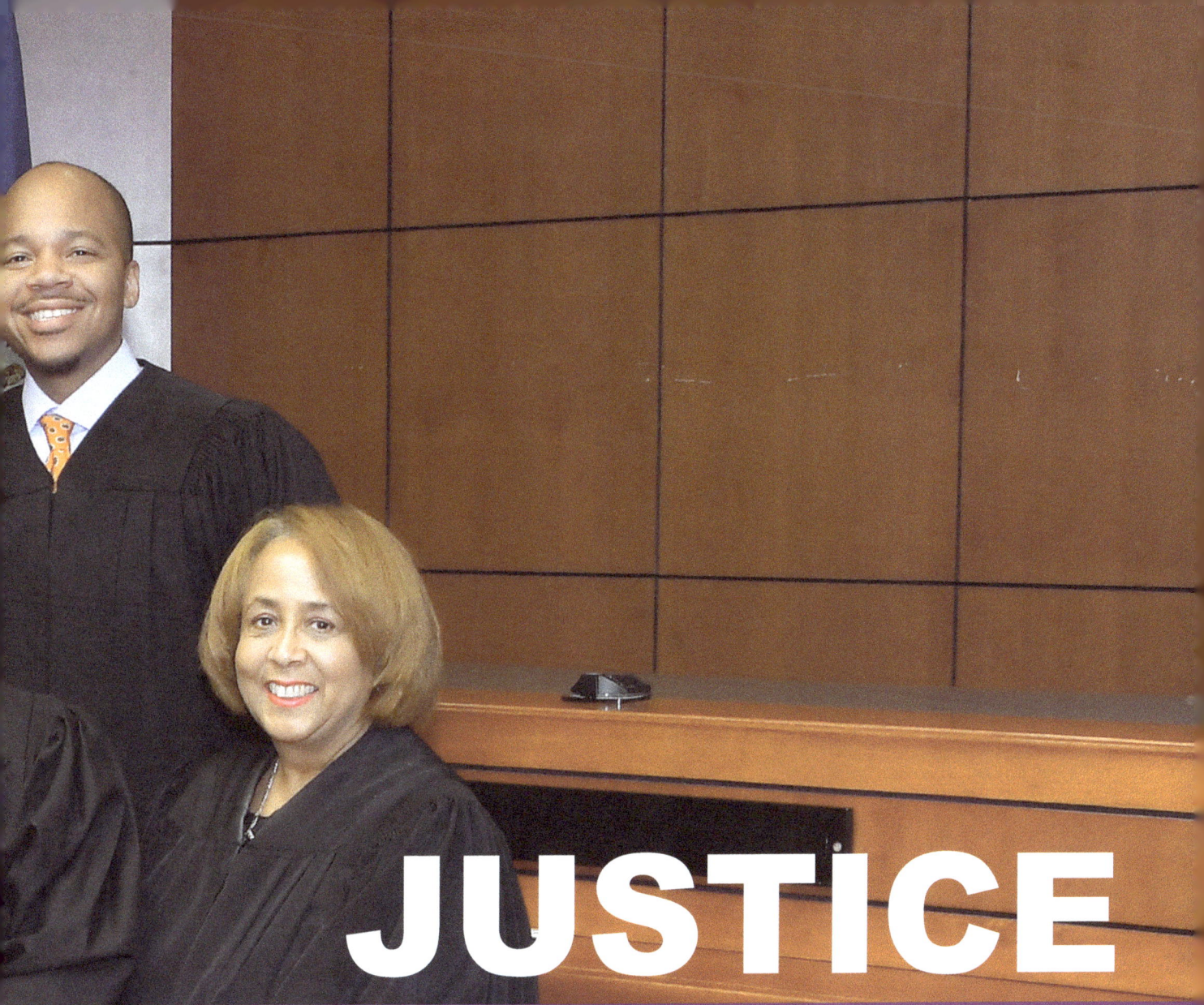

JUSTICE

We must be concerned with massive incarceration in our state, where African Americans are 8.3% of the commonwealth's total population, but are approximately 29% of Kentucky's prison population.[26] The effects of disproportionate incarceration, racially-motivated policing strategies, and racially-biased discriminatory and mandatory sentencing should all be thoroughly studied in our city. After which, a plan of action should be instituted that will reduce incarceration and improve community safety. People of color receive harsher penalties, more jail time, and are treated more aggressively and with considerably more force than their White counterparts by law enforcement agents.[27] [28]

We must urge local law enforcement to review and update performance-based standards to ensure that incidents of misconduct will be minimized through appropriate management, training, and oversight protocols and, when such incidents occur, they are properly investigated. We must seek to provide police officers with the tools to work in our communities to enhance their professional growth and education. We must give power to local communities over agencies, who have a responsibility to "protect and serve" by supporting the establishment of independent civilian

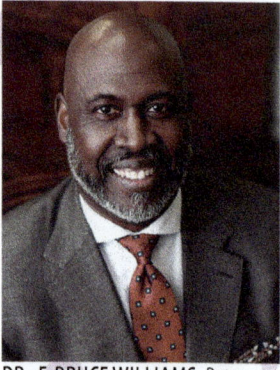

DR. F. BRUCE WILLIAMS, Bates Memorial Baptist Church

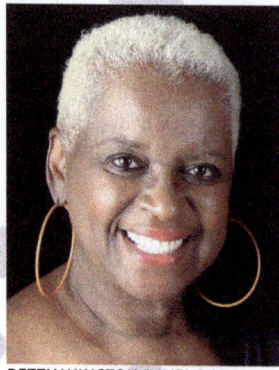

BETTY WINSTON BAYE', Columnist

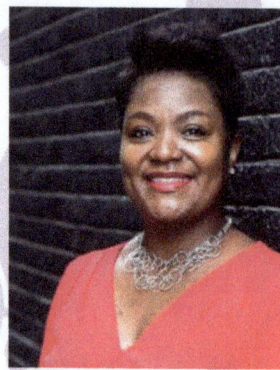

SADIQA N. REYNOLDS, ESQ., Louisville Urban League

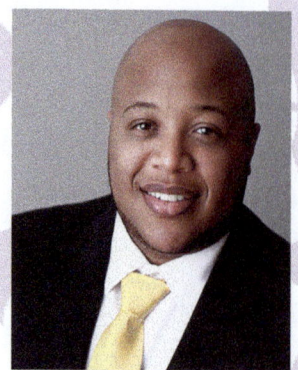

KEVIN COWHERD, Kentuckians For The Commonwealth

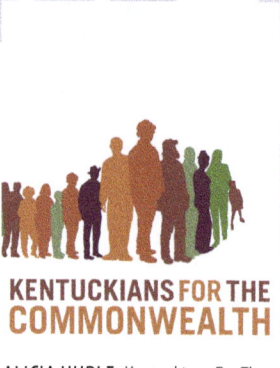

ALICIA HURLE, Kentuckians For The Commonwealth

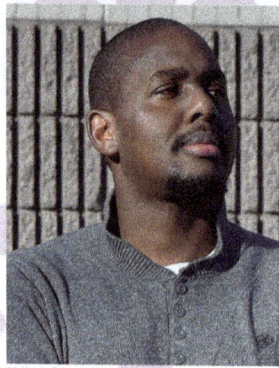

LYNDON PRYOR, Louisville Urban League

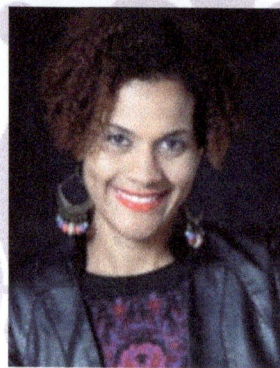

DR. CHERIE DAWSON-EDWARDS, University of Louisville

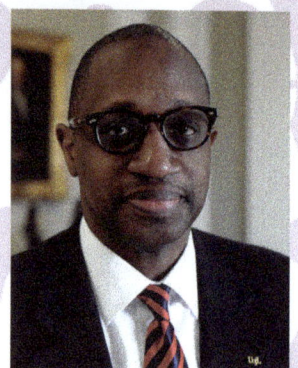

CEDRIC MERLIN POWELL, University of Louisville

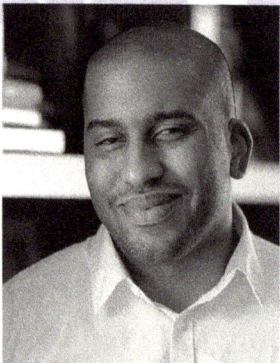

DORIAN O. BURTON, William R. Kenan, Jr. Charitable Trust

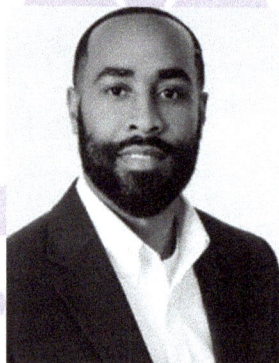

BRIAN C.B. BARNES, Tennessee Achievement School District

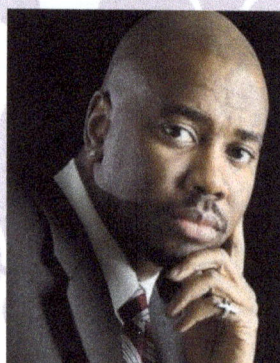

DR. RICKY L. JONES, University of Louisville

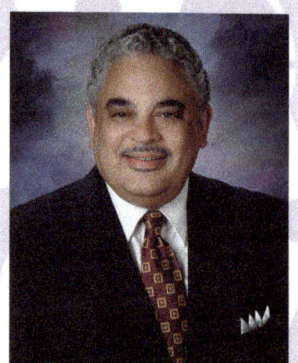

JOHN J. JOHNSON, Kentucky Commission on Human Rights

review boards that are reflective of the racial and ethnic makeup of the community.

Further, as a community we must take a proactive approach to steer at-risk youth away from gangs and toward being successful, productive members of the community. We must support prevention and intervention that direct our youth in the right direction.

John J. Johnson, Executive Director
Kentucky Commission on Human Rights

THE EVANGELICAL CHURCH: TURNING A BLIND EYE TO RACIAL INJUSTICE

Dr. F. Bruce Williams, Pastor
Bates Memorial Baptist Church

One of the reasons racism and white supremacy has persisted in America is because it has historically garnered support and justification for its existence from various corners of American life. It was necessary for America to find ways to justify the continued existence of white supremacy not only to maintain power and privilege, but also because you cannot treat people with such damnable inhumanity and maintain your own sense of humanity. So, white America has historically turned to disciplines like science, biology, and psychology to help support White supremacy. One institution that has been complicit in this is the white evangelical church in America.

The white evangelical church in America has historically been guilty of providing the system of white supremacy and racism with the theological underpinnings necessary to justify its existence and persistence. Racist teachings like "the curse of Ham" were among many teachings that helped justify

and promote institutions like slavery, Jim and Jane Crow laws, and a host of other expressions of white supremacy designed to maintain power and privilege for whites in America. This is because its parishioners have been the beneficiaries of the privileges inherent in being white in a system that favors whites.

Unfortunately, this is one of the main reasons why the white evangelical church, as a whole, has not participated in promoting justice in American society. It has, in fact, been an obstacle to justice in American life. It may claim the truth housed in our national documents: "We hold these truths to be self evident, that all men are created equal....", but any real struggle to make that truth a reality in American life has been met with either the church's resistance or silence.

As a consequence, the evangelical church has persistently been on the wrong side of history when it comes to the struggle for justice. It has been at odds with a church tradition that produced the likes of Nat Turner, Denmark Vesey, Sojourner Truth, Frederick Douglass, Martin Luther King, Jr. and a host other of men and women, clergy, and lay people, whose passion for justice was fueled by their Christian faith. This justice tradition often noted the hypocrisy of the evangelical church and rejected its racist theology and its complicity with white supremacy.

Sadly, the evangelical church has routinely turned a blind eye to racism and a deaf ear to the call for racial justice. The election of Donald Trump by over 80% of evangelicals is an example of this. It is telling how the evangelical church seemed to completely ignore the racist (as well as misogynistic, xenophobic, and homophobic) verbiage and history of discrimination attributed to Donald Trump in order to put him in office. Some would even argue that it was, in fact, Trump's racist verbiage and backward glance to the racist good ole days housed in his campaign slogan to "Make America Great Again" that appealed to the core of the evangelical church.

Too often evangelicals seem to think that Christianity has to do with personal piety but has nothing to do with justice. This deficient theological and biblical thinking reveals a disconnect between how they see one's relationship with God and its connection to one's relationship to others. On one occasion, Jesus made it clear that the two greatest commandments are to love God with all of your heart... and your neighbor as yourself. On these two, he said, hangs all of the law and the prophets (Matthew 22:36-40).

[37] ...'Love the Lord your God with all your heart and with all your soul and with all your mind.' [38] This is the first and greatest commandment. [39] And the second is like it: 'Love your neighbor as yourself.' [40] All the Law and the Prophets hang on these two commandments."

-Matthew 22: 37-40 (NIV)

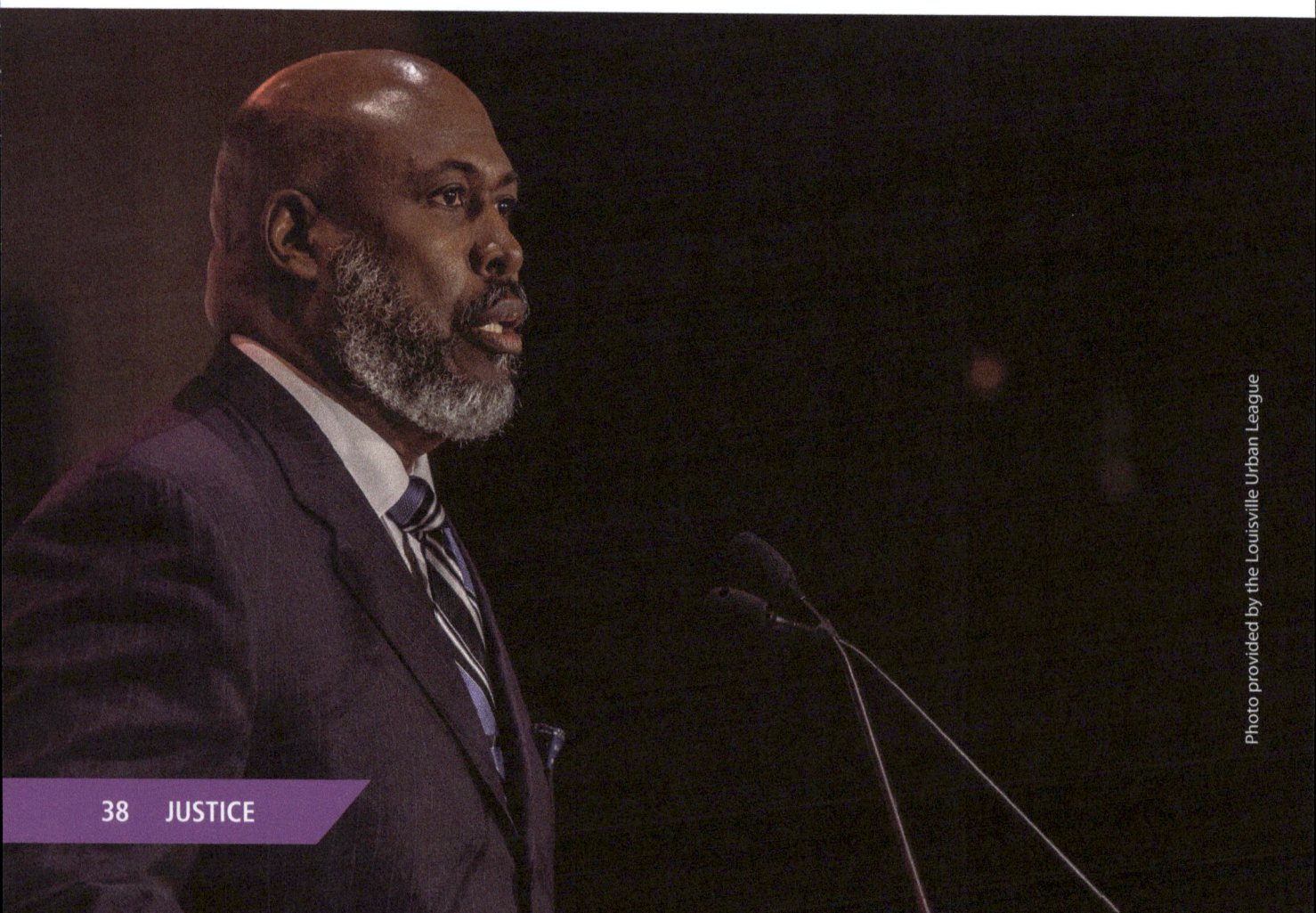

These commandments describe both the vertical and horizontal relationships central to Christianity, which are inextricably bound together. You cannot claim to love a God you have never seen and mistreat your brother and sister whom you see all the time (1 John 4:20). So these two relationships are never independent of one another. If justice involves treating others the way you will want to be treated and the way God wants you to treat them, then it stands to reason that if you are a Christian, tied to your relationship to God is how you relate to other fellow human beings. But if you promote personal piety and forget that it is tied to your relationship to others, then you are missing what it means to be a follower of Jesus.

Evangelicals seem to have a disconnect there. Or if they do connect the two, they want justice (just relationships) without paying the cost. They want racial reconciliation without paying the price. How can that be if your theology insists that a price had to be paid for you to be reconciled to God? If reconciliation costs, then evangelicals need to be prepared to pay the cost for racial reconciliation. The problem is they want the benefit without the payment. To paraphrase Frederick Douglass, they want rain without thunder and lightening, crops without tilling the soil, the beauty of the ocean without the mighty roar of its many waters.[29] Justice in America requires a radical reordering of American society and a radical sharing of power. And there are no calls for *that* from the evangelical church.

Justice costs. Justice requires change. But evangelicals seem more concerned about maintaining "order" than bringing about justice. That is why "law and order" rhetoric seems so appealing to the evangelical church. They value "law and order". To them, what's legal equals what's right. But everything that's legal is not right. Slavery was legal. Jim Crow was legal. Apartheid in South Africa was legal. Redlining and discrimination in housing was legal. Just because something is legal does not mean it's right. Dr. King declared that an unjust law is no

law at all.[30] You cannot have true peace without true justice. No justice, no peace.

Turning a blind eye to justice is to turn a blind eye to those who suffer from injustice. And to ignore them is to ignore Jesus...

If the evangelical church is going to be true to its founder, then it must open its eyes to racial injustice and be prepared to pay the cost to make it real. If it is going to promote racial reconciliation, then it cannot be done without addressing the issue of justice. This means that in order for there to be true racial reconciliation, the white evangelical church will have to confess the sin of racism, repent (which is more than offering letters of apology; to repent means to change your behavior), repair damages done by racism (this is called reparations), and commit to the continued struggle for justice, understanding that promoting justice is a vital part of what it means to promote the Kingdom of God and its King.

Turning a blind eye to justice is to turn a blind eye to those who suffer from injustice. And to ignore them is to ignore Jesus, for Jesus said, "When you've done it to the least of these...you've done it also unto me" (Matthew 25:35-45).

KILLING US SOFTLY: BLACKS DO NOT GET THE SAME PORTRAYAL IN THE MEDIA AS WHITES

Betty Winston Baye', Columnist, Author, Motivational Speaker

TV One's cancellation of Roland Martin's "NewsOne Now" is a terrible loss to those who thirst for an unapologetically Black perspective on the news. Martin's was the only Black daily newscast on television, and the last of serious daily news shows that focused on issues related to Black people. Meanwhile, Black magazines and newspapers are also struggling to retain readers and advertisers as more African Americans join the great migration to social media.

In this heated media environment, Black organizations must take to digital and social media with a vengeance. And when the best interests of Black people happen to coincide with the interests of others, healthy collaborations should be explored.

Procter & Gamble, for example, launched its "My Black Is Beautiful" campaign at the urging of Black women within the company who wanted "to help redefine beauty standards." Last summer, the household,

feminine, beauty and health products company released "The Talk." The two-minute video depicted Black mothers schooling their children on how to handle racial slurs; being excluded from a game because they're Black; and how to survive a routine traffic stop.

P&G's video echoed a passage from Dr. Martin Luther King Jr.'s 1963 "Letter from Birmingham Jail." King described the angst of a having to "suddenly find your tongue twisted and your speech stammering as you seek to explain to your six-year-old daughter why she can't go to the public amusement park that has just been advertised on television, and see tears welling up in her eyes when she is told that Funtown is closed to colored children, and see ominous clouds of inferiority beginning to form in her little mental sky, and see her beginning to distort her personality by developing an unconscious bitterness toward White people…".

Critics attacked P&G's video as anti-White, anti-police, and "identity politics pandering." Michelle Malkin, or "Ann Coulter lite" as I call her, lit into the ad in the National Review, calling it "propaganda," aimed at "the social justice crowd," as if social justice is offensive.[31] P&G "should stick to selling diapers instead of filling them," she wrote, as if she, the American-born daughter of Filipino immigrants and who is married to a White man is, of course, an expert on the lived experiences of generations of African Americans.

It's true that America's "Funtowns" are now open to all with money to pay and "Whites only" signs are in museums, but those changes came because good people – Black and White – marched, bled, went to jail, and died, and because brave journalists exposed the horrors behind "Cotton Curtain."

America elected a Black president *twice,* but how much would you wager that even Barack and Michelle Obama have felt obliged to give their two very privileged daughters "The Talk." It's irresponsible not to prepare Black children for racism. The point isn't to burden them, but to enlighten and strengthen their resolve to push back. Racism is a form of bullying. You don't need to have "The Talk" if your children get so much positive feedback in school, in the media, and from society at-large about their looks, their smarts, and their potential.

Much of the fear and loathing Black people experience is fueled by local media's outsized emphasis on Black pathology. Black criminals are far too often depicted over Black achievers, as if Black pathology is the norm and black achievement is the exception. The persistent and overwhelmingly negative portrayals of Black people impacts how they are perceived by others. Even worse, it impacts how Black people perceive themselves. How are Black children to believe they are smart, beautiful, capable, and act accordingly when multiple times almost daily the news media show their neighborhoods as devastated, their schools as failing, their parents as broken, and their people in mug shots and being carted off in shackles and cuffs?

Incessant repetition has psychological consequences. If your worldview is shaped by a corrosive narrative which suggests that Black lives don't matter – not even your own – or that your life choices narrow down to jail or death, what's the point of living? Crime news is cheap to produce, which is why resource-starved local media deliver so much of it.

Donald Trump has tweeted that Black people were responsible for 81% of the killings of White people.

That was a lie.

Politifact, a nonpartisan fact-checking website, gave Trump its highest "pants on fire" rating for that.[32] The FBI's uniform crime-reporting data for 2016 indicated that 89.5% of Black victims of homicide were killed by other Blacks and 81.6% of White victims were killed by other Whites.[33]

So if most homicides and violent victimizations are intra-racial, why do media rarely refer to "White-on-White crime"?

The Root online magazine's Michael Harriot reported out the federal Bureau of Justice Statistics findings that "less than 1% of Blacks overall (about 2% of Black men) commit a violent crime in any given year."[34] Harriot's article ran under the cheeky headline, "Why We Never Talk About Black-on-Black Crime: An Answer to White America's Most Pressing Question."

Black people, of course, notice the discrepancies in news coverage that helps to perpetuate the notion that we are somehow criminal by nature while Whites who murder – including White mass murderers – are just misguided souls, certainly not domestic terrorists, and assuredly not representative of White pathology.

Black people noticed the TIME Magazine cover of O.J. Simpson, with his complexion darkened considerably.

The altered photo of the retired football star was published atop the headline "An American Tragedy" while Simpson was on trial accused of murdering his White ex-wife and her friend.

Black people notice that when the targets were Black substance abusers, the media ran with government's fearsome declaration of "a war on drugs." Yet, now when the targeted abusers are primarily White, the government isn't at war. It's engaged in a more civilized-sounding, "opioid interdiction" in response to a "crisis" to help people who are not criminals needing to be jailed, but who are "sick" and in need of treatment and the public's compassion.

Meanwhile, had it not been for Black voters, especially women, Alabama might have elected an alleged pedophile to the U.S. Senate in late 2017. The media were caught short by the Black wave because in the run up to the election, they focused almost exclusively on White women and the White vote. Again, the media played Black people cheap and they noticed.

New York Times columnist Nicholas Kristof noted that the media tend to "cover planes that crash, not those that take off and land safely."[35] That's a good summary of how Black America is covered by the media: our plane takeoffs seem to not to get coverage. All we see are plane crashes, but we've got lots of planes taking off. There are wonderful things going on in our community. We know our success stories and we talk about our celebrations, but who reports it? After years of inaccurately painting a community a certain way, then that's what society at-large will see the community as.

Unless there's a media paradigm shift, new generations of Black children, their mental skies polluted by noxious clouds of inferiority, will arise and ask not only as Dr. King mentioned, "Daddy, why do White people treat colored people so mean" but "Why do Black people treat other Black people so mean?"

FIXES WILL TAKE PRAYER AND PEN

Sadiqa N. Reynolds, Esq., President and CEO
Louisville Urban League

The Louisville Urban League supports the idea of corporate prayer coupled with corporate investment. God can do His part, but He wants us to meet Him halfway. The governor, with his mighty pen, must change broken policy, must use his time with the President of the United States to assist in helping "the least of these."

God will be honored when leaders do their work. Depending on his heart, a governor that prays is a good thing, but praying while promulgating policy that kills and destroys does not honor God. Faith is necessary, but faith without works is dead.

Here are some ideas for the work we'd like to see the governor take on in partnership with other elected officials:

- ▶ Illegal guns should be destroyed when the police get them. Change the law that prevents that.

- ▶ Dilapidated school buildings should be repaired before any government spends a dime on building or supporting a charter school.

- ▶ Communities that have been historically redlined out of economic opportunity should be strategically invested in with community input.

- ▶ Gap financing should be made available to support homeownership, so that poor communities can begin wealth building.

- ▶ Also, go ahead and pay for universal pre-K. We have the data to show that this a big game changer.

- ▶ Let's require that the percentage of minorities on a construction job reflect the percentage of minorities in that community. Also, declare that they must, in fact, be from that community and not Louisiana, Georgia, or elsewhere. At the very least, make the city and state training programs priority for hiring.

God will be honored when leaders do their work.

▶ Please make sure people have access to affordable health care. We can call it Bevincare, Trumpcare or anything other than Obamacare, but don't be a part of taking it away. We know it needs to be fixed, but the fix should cover more people, not fewer.

▶ Require that every developer building housing in our state set aside a certain amount of that housing for affordable housing. Let's deconstruct the idea of concentrating poverty.

▶ Treat Black drug addicts with the compassion and humanity with which you treat the drug addicts in your own family. We could have saved entire communities with what we are now spending on Narcan. Our police are reviving some people twice in a day because life is valuable and worth saving. Show us that you love God and that our lives are valuable too.

So, we will continue to pray, but we will be working hard and ask that you would do the same. We want the violence to end and we believe it requires us to deal with past ills and painful policy.

BLACK POLITICAL POWER AND CIVIC ENGAGEMENT

Alicia Hurle, Deputy Organizing Director for Democracy
Kevin Cowherd, Grassroots Leader
Kentuckians For The Commonwealth

After Reconstruction, most Southern states instituted legal barriers to voting for Black citizens. However, Kentucky lawmakers did not seek to pass state legislation to deny black Kentuckians the right to vote. This may have been due to the relatively small Black population in the commonwealth and the assumption that they were not a significant political threat to the status quo. However, in larger cities like Louisville with an ever-growing Black population, Black voters were able to weld increasing political power beginning in the early 20th century.

An early example of Black political power in Louisville was in 1917, when Black voters aligned with the Republican Party to help restore the party's control in Louisville. At this point in history, Black voters supported Republicans candidates and the party courted black voters to further their loyalty to the party. In the 1920s, Black Louisville residents formed the Lincoln Independent Party in an attempt to shift support of Black voters. The party did not win any

elections, but they did manage to convince the city's Republican administration to hire its first Black city employees.[36]

Under President Franklin Roosevelt, the Democratic Party began to attract support from Black voters across the country. As Black voters in the state shifted their support, for the first time there was a competition for the Black vote in Kentucky.

In 1935, Charles W. Anderson of Louisville was elected to the state legislature. He was the first Black Kentuckian elected to statewide office since Reconstruction. During his time in Frankfort, Anderson and the Black legislators from Louisville who followed in his footsteps, were able to introduce legislation that dismantled legal segregation in Kentucky.

Back home in Louisville, White flight from the city into the suburbs beginning in the 1930s led to increased

Black voting power in Louisville. Black representation on the Louisville Board of Aldermen rose from 8% in 1945 to 33% in the 1980s. In fact, in the early 1980s, Joe Hammond and other Black Louisville leaders created PAC-10, a Black political action committee that raised money to support Black candidates running for local offices like county commissioner.

The number of Black elected officials in Louisville has receded somewhat in recent years. There are currently four Black legislators representing Jefferson County, including Representative Attica Scott, who in 2016 was the first Black woman elected to the state legislature in nearly 20 years. After the Louisville Board of Alderman gave way to the Louisville Metro County following city/county merger in 2003, Black representation within this citywide elected body fell from 33% to 23%. And following the 2016 election, only five of 26 (or 19%) Metro Council members were Black.[37]

This is an under-representation considering that

Black people make up approximately 22% of the Metro Louisville population.[38] There is one Black school board member – Diane Porter – who became the first Black woman elected to chair the Jefferson County Board of Education in 2012, which is also a feat she has since accomplished again. There is also some Black representation on several municipal city councils. However, as reported in 2016, only 18% of Metro Louisville Board and Commission positions are held by Black Louisvillians.[39]

There are several Black-led civic organizations in Louisville that: promote civic participation; host political education events; host candidate forums and debates; and organize voter registration, education, and mobilization efforts. Examples include the Louisville Urban League, Black Lives Matter Louisville, NAACP Louisville Branch, Kentucky Alliance Against Racist and Political Repression, and several Black fraternity and sorority chapters. Politicians and parties continue to compete for Black votes during elections. In fact, voters in Louisville continue have

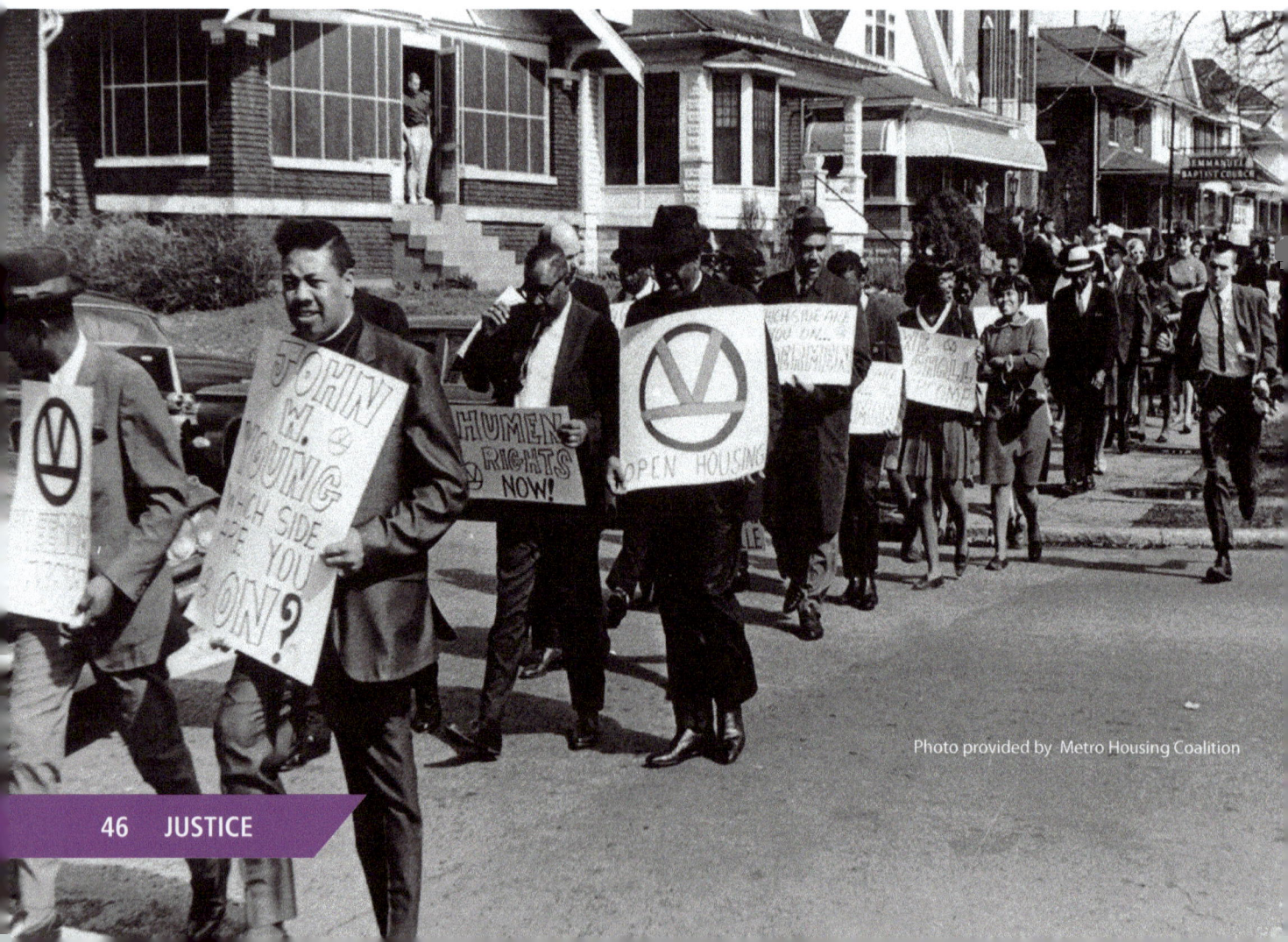

Photo provided by Metro Housing Coalition

the power to swing major local, state, and federal elections in Kentucky. However, voter turnout in Louisville continues to be low in predominately Black communities.

In addition, one in four voting-age, Black Kentuckians are barred from voting because they have been convicted of a felony.[40] Felony disenfranchisement was enshrined in the Kentucky Constitution in 1891 and began having a significant impact on Black Kentuckians in the age of mass incarceration. In fact, Kentucky has the highest Black disenfranchisement rate in the country and is only one of four permanent disenfranchisement states.[41]

POLICY RECOMMENDATIONS

1. Organize a statewide effort to increase voting access for Black Kentuckians:

   ▶ Black-led civic organizations can continue to work with allied groups on a unified advocacy strategy and grassroots campaign to pass a Restoration of Voting Rights Bill in the state legislature and win the proceeding ballot measure. Victory means that felony disenfranchisement is eradicated in Kentucky and 26% of Black Kentuckians regain their voting rights without being required to go through an expungement process. Examples of allied groups include Kentucky Council of Churches, Kentuckians For The Commonwealth, Louisville Showing Up for Racial Justice, Kentucky Jobs with Justice, and UFCW Local 227. These non-

   ▶ Black-led organizations advocate for policies, such as the restoration of voting rights for former felons in Kentucky, that will have positive impacts on the Black community and/or do civic engagement work in Black communities.

   ▶ Black-led civic organizations can work with allied groups to advocate for increased voter

access in Kentucky via measures like same-day or automatic voter registration, accessible polling locations, longer polling hours, early voting, and less stringent voter identification policies.

2. Black-led civic organizations can work together to create a Black candidate pipeline by organizing formalized recruitment efforts and candidate trainings, as well as offering support to Black candidates running for local, state, and federal offices and seeking appointments on local boards and commissions.

3. Black-led civic organizations can band together to organize voter engagement efforts in the Black community that goes beyond traditional voter registration and Get Out the Vote drives. These efforts can include:

   ▶ Ongoing political education and engagement in the Black community

   ▶ Opportunities for intergenerational sharing and learning about Louisville's Black political history

   ▶ Inclusive spaces for Black leaders of various backgrounds to work together to create and mobilize around a political agenda that seeks to improve the quality of life for all Black Louisvillians.

THERE IS NO FENCE TO SIT ON

Sadiqa N. Reynolds, Esq., President and CEO
Lyndon Pryor, Director of Health Education and Policy
Louisville Urban League

There are many in favor of the preservation of Confederate monuments in the public square. On the other side are those adamantly against their positions of honor and prestige in the public eye. There is much to say about both groups, but those attempting to position themselves in the middle are most intriguing, as they claim positions of neutrality or faux objectivity in the name of "seeing both sides."

We challenge those proverbial fence sitters. This position, when placed in the context of historical fact, does not hold water. Plainly put – there is no middle ground.

When it comes to issues of race and racism, the ugly history of slavery, and the heinous institutions, policies, and practices it birthed, there is no middle ground. In August and September of 2017, there were particularly a lot of heated discussions about the placement and position of old relics of the Confederacy across our country. Contrary to the accusations of many opponents to the removal of the statues, this fight is not at all new.

Protests against Confederate trophies can be traced to the 1800s when White and Black Union veterans objected to the inclusion of Confederate graves in Memorial Day celebrations.

In 1869, the White Union Adjutant General William T. Collins, wrote, "We strew flowers on the graves of our comrades, and prevent their being strewn in the national cemeteries at the same time, on graves of such rebel dead as may be buried therein… because we seek to mark in this distinction and manner the feelings with which the nation regards freedom and slavery, loyalty and treason… mere courage never ennobled treason. It cannot turn slavery into liberty, or make despotic intentions desirable and to-be-applauded virtues. Our refusal to decorate rebel graves marks… our undying hostility to the ideas for which they fought and died. To do less than keep this

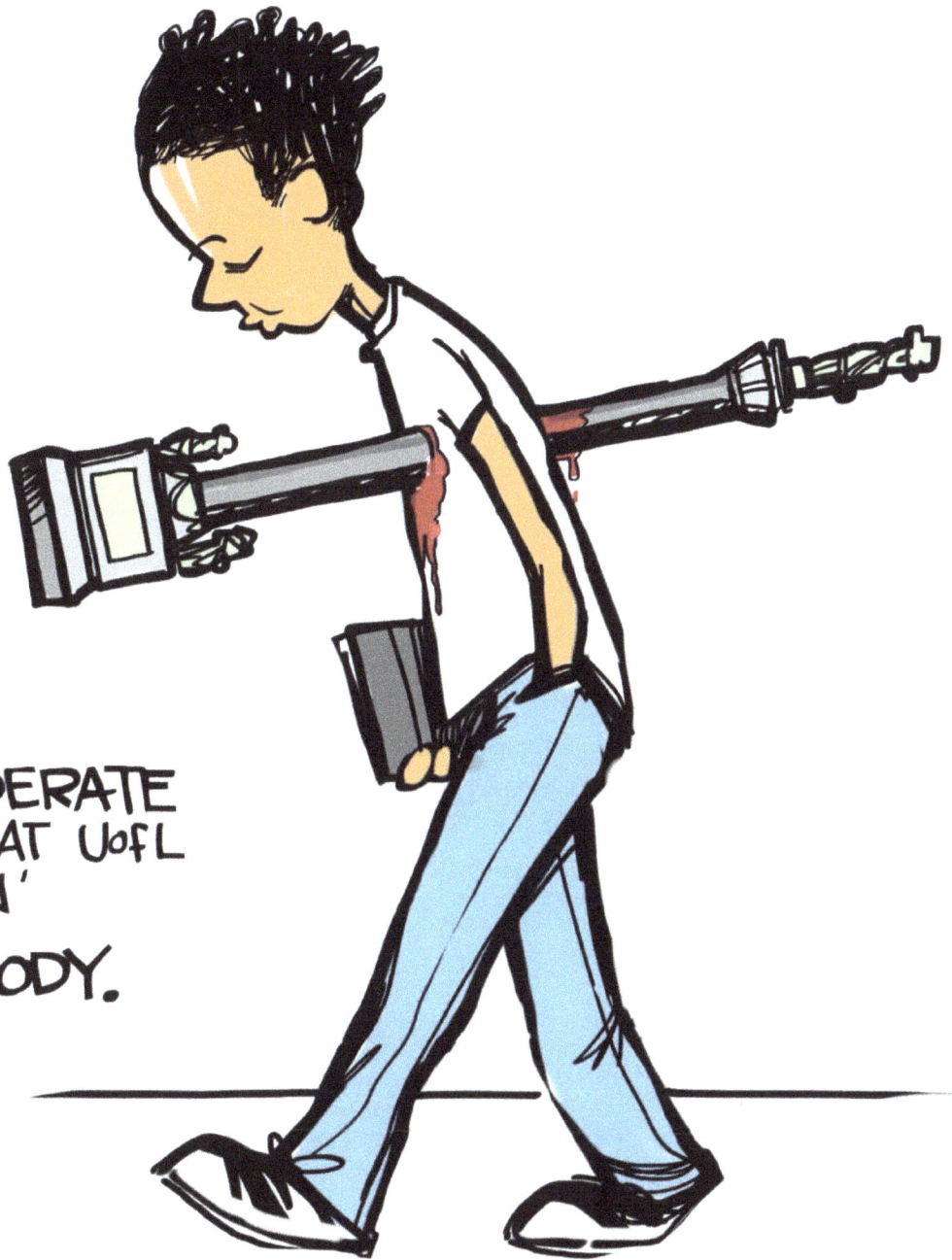

THAT CONFEDERATE STATUE OVER AT UofL AIN'T HURTIN' NOBODY.

distinction fresh in the national mind is to undermine the republic itself."[42]

For years, African Americans have objected to the construction of monuments and use of flags and other symbols. However, we learned from the murder of Viola Gregg Liuzzo, the White civil rights activist killed by the Ku Klux Klan in 1965, it sometimes takes a tragedy of just the right hue for people to pay attention.

You are either for continued celebration and honor of those who fought and died, or were willing to die, for the right to systematically subjugate, brutalize and murder an entire race of people based solely on their skin color and desire for wealth or you are not.

A modern example is the response to the heroin epidemic. Historically, the response to addiction was jail, but the response changes as the hue of the addict changes. Police are now armed with Narcan, and money for life-saving treatment seems unlimited. It seems we can't calculate the value of life until we know the race of the victim. Thus, we understand that the statues stand as evidence that the victims of the atrocities committed are not valued by their country.

Your silence or ambivalence on this issue does not make you fair, impartial, or well-reasoned. Your willingness to "discuss" the merits of removal with both sides or take into consideration the perspectives of those most affected – as if our lived experiences are up for debate – makes you neither compassionate nor emotionally intelligent.

Rather, they call attention to your disregard for the emotional and literal harm they inflict on generations.

No one, we are familiar with, in favor of the removal of Confederate statues from the public square, is in favor of erasing these monsters from history. In fact, we are staunch advocates for the teaching of a complete American history – a history that includes the atrocities committed against Native Americans, the transatlantic slave trade, the Civil War, Reconstruction, the dismantling of Reconstruction, Jim Crow, segregation, the prison industrial complex, and more.

We want history preserved and told because we must learn from it. But monuments are not necessary for learning and truth.

We need more substantive engagement in museums, books, documentaries, theaters and classrooms.

Monuments honoring losers teach us that there are not consequences for actions, however heinous they may be, particularly (and this is most painful) when the victim is Black. They teach us that our darkest moments as a nation should be celebrated. Worst of all, they teach us to forget that the victims of the perpetrators we honor are still here and suffering from that trauma daily.

This debate is not about statues, but who and whose values get valued. It is about how we continue to respond or not, to today's discrimination, hate, and marginalization and how symbols reflect our behavior, our values, our endorsement.

Where you fall is a matter of personal conscience, but you must choose. Jefferson Davis said, "You cannot transform the negro into anything one-tenth as useful or as good as what slavery enables him to be."[43] If you are neutral on whether a monument to him in the Capitol rotunda stays or goes… you have indeed chosen a side, because there is no fence to sit on.

DISRUPTING LOUISVILLE'S SCHOOL-TO-PRISON PIPELINE THROUGH RESTORATIVE JUSTICE

Dr. Cherie Dawson-Edwards

Anne Braden Institute for Social Justice Research, University of Louisville

While they make up only 29% of the population, Black youth are 74% of youth detained in Louisville.[44] A 2014 report found that Black youth in Jefferson County were more likely to be adjudicated delinquent, arrested, and detained in Department of Juvenile Justice facilities, while less likely to receive probation.[45] The same report recommended that Kentucky counties experiencing racial disparities in their juvenile justice process should "Adopt restorative approaches, rooted in addressing diversity issues throughout the juvenile justice continuum,"

Restorative justice practices focus on repairing harm by including the offender, victim, and community in resolving conflict.[46] Louisville is the first city in Kentucky to have a restorative justice alternative in the court process for youth. Restorative Justice Louisville (RJL) is "a collaborative effort between legal professionals and members of our community working together to promote the use of RJ practices in our judicial system."[47] The program served its first youth in March 2011 beginning in the Louisville Metro Police Department 2nd Division, and now includes the 1st and 4th Divisions. RJL costs $1,014 per case compared to community supervision ($3, 166 per case) and incarceration ($42,542 per youth).[48]

The most recent RJL update reveals some interesting findings about how they are serving individuals from diverse backgrounds. They found that Black victims are less likely to participate in restorative justice compared to Whites.[49] As it relates to youth involved in the system, RJL reported that 62% were Black and most of the youth referred to RJL come from West Louisville. Offense type also differed by race: Black youth have more property offense referrals at almost double the rate of White youth.

While restorative justice has seen some successes in the justice system, its corollary for schools – restorative practices – has also been widely successful in cities such as San Francisco, Oakland, and Denver.

Some restorative justice advocates suggest that it is "best applied to the educational domain, rather than the criminal justice system…[because] school community members see each other daily and even minor encounters can easily turn dangerous if not handled adequately," (p. 540).[50]

In Louisville, the 2013 Jefferson County Public Schools (JCPS) Equity Scorecard showed serious disproportionality issues in school suspension and achievement across the district.[51] As a result of the Scorecard, several substantive changes were made to the 2014 JCPS Code of Acceptable Behavior, including a revised Restorative Practices (RP) policy. Over the next two years, the Department of Diversity, Equity and Poverty Programs (DEP) sponsored district-wide professional development trainings to over 700 JCPS stakeholders, including principals, assistant principals, counselors, School Response Teams (SRTs), Positive Behavior Intervention Supports (PBIS) school leads, and teachers. As more district stakeholders become familiar with the philosophy,

the potential for restorative practices as a proactive strategy that complements other district-wide initiatives, like Positive Behavior Intervention Supports (PBIS), became apparent. Currently, the district is aligning restorative practices initiatives with PBIS schools.

District research has long shown that placement in alternative school leads to a higher probability of children entering into the justice system. A study published in 2015 found that almost 40% of JCPS students placed in alternative school experience subsequent juvenile detention.[52] They also found that 50% of Black students experience alternative school placement compared to 32% of white students. When considering race and gender together, both Black girls and boys were overrepresented in both alternative school placement and subsequent juvenile detention.

In 2015, JCPS leadership created Minor Daniels Academy (MDA), a middle-high behavioral alternative

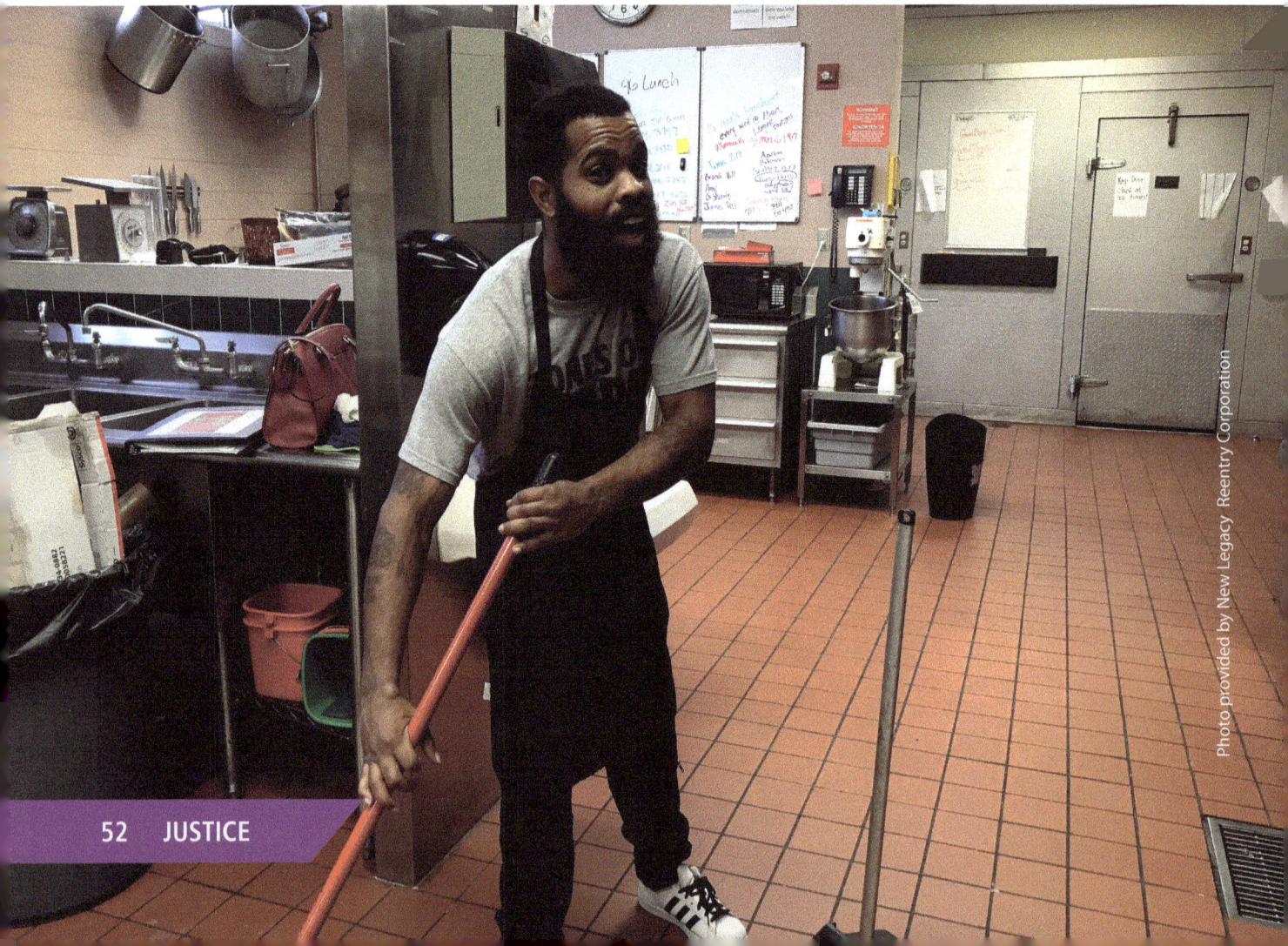

school. Currently, there are 189 students attending MDA. Ninety-two percent of the students are Black - 55% Black males and 37% Black females. The school's opening was marred with negative press and questioned about its representation as a "restorative academy". However, with the support of JCPS Department of Diversity, Poverty and Equity Programs, MDA staff immediately set a plan to implement restorative practices throughout the school. Starting with counselors and other administrators, MDA began its path to creating a restorative culture by establishing their needs and preferred outcomes. During the next two years, the school rolled out restorative practices implementation through a professional learning community and various trainings. By the end of their second school year, MDA became the first JCPS school to consistently use restorative practices strategies, such as nonviolent communication, restorative circles, and informal conferencing.

Based on data collected in 2016, the staff held approximately 60 community-building circles per grading period.[53] Now it is common to see teachers using circles for learning and for morning check-in. While MDA is in its third year of restorative practices implementation, other schools are just beginning the process. The district allotted $2.3 million to fund the Behavioral Support Systems Team in their efforts to integrate Positive Behavior Intervention Supports and Restorative Practices in more schools. While restorative practices is a philosophy, in JCPS, it is also a specific strategy falling under Behavior Supports. The first cohort is comprised of 18 schools that will receive training, support, and resources from the International Institute for Restorative Practices (IIRP).

In order to disrupt the school-to-prison pipeline, methods addressing youth behavioral concerns should steer away from the binary procedures outlined in zero tolerance or "tough on crime" practices and move toward programs like those of positive behavioral change, treatment, and restorative justice practices for our young people.

More specifically, we need to:

▶ Develop a clear and inclusive definition of RJP for Louisville.

▶ Equip parents and community members with the tools to advocate for the use of RJP in the justice system and schools.

▶ Train community groups to conduct restorative justice practices in the most affected communities.

▶ Hold elected officials (Metro Government and the JCPS School Board) accountable for ensuring that funded RJP programs prioritize addressing disparities in our school and justice systems.

RENAME AIRPORT AFTER MUHAMMAD ALI

Sadiqa N. Reynolds, Esq., President and CEO
Louisville Urban League

Among many things to prepare for as you consider naming or renaming a building, on every list is controversy. We certainly don't need unnecessary controversy as there is plenty happening in the world without intentionally stirring it up. So given that warning, I've considered this idea and still find no legitimate reason why it shouldn't be done.

What's the "it"?

There have been conversations in our city about changing the name of Louisville International Airport to the "Muhammad Ali International Airport," and that is an idea that we can get behind. Certainly, Ali was a favorite son of the city and we've all seen the stats and surveys that showed he was repeatedly among the most well-known figures in the world, even being called one of "The 20 Most Influential Americans of All Time" by TIME Magazine.[54]

Of course, fame alone is no reason to honor a person with the naming of an airport. After all, there are many people who are famous for foolish and sundry endeavors. So, most would agree that we should wait to judge a person's whole life before we sign over naming rights.

It is time. We know his story. We know it all. The great, the good, and the ugly.

In fact, he is one of the few public figures loved by people that might disagree with him religiously, romantically, and philosophically. His life was lived transparently. He was forced to declare his God, and he did. Whatever you believe about his beliefs, the idea that a man would risk life, limb, and freedom to peacefully stand loyal is worth honoring.

And in fact, we have honored him along with the rest of the world.

I have asked many, and it is hard, if not impossible, to name another time that our country has seemed to pause and stand together in the way that we did during the service honoring the life of Ali. Of course, we have come together during tragedies forever engrained in our hearts and minds, but the time we spent honoring his life was a time of great celebration. Rarely does the death of any person bring the world together in the way that Ali's death did. Surely this is because of the life he lived. He stood for the principles that are now embodied in the Muhammad Ali Center: confidence, conviction, dedication, giving, respect, spirituality.

Ali has been the recipient of more awards than we have space to list, including the Lifetime Achievement Award given by Amnesty International, as well as being named "International Ambassador" of Jubilee 2000, a global organization.

And what is most special about Ali is that while he belongs to the world, he is first the son of Louisville. Any familial ties begin in this city, blocks from the Louisville Urban League and a short car ride from the Louisville International Airport.

Who better to honor with the renaming of our airport? He is a symbol of what our city is aspiring to be. We strive to be a city where race doesn't matter, religion doesn't matter, and who you love is not a barrier. We are not there, but having his name so

prominently placed would remind us each day of what our aspirations are. This is not to suggest that he was perfect; he was not. However, if we judge him by human standards, he was a giant among men – not simply because he was a great boxer, not just because he stood up for himself, but because of the way he loved us… all of us.

He saw beyond skin color, nation of origin, religion, and other differences often used to divide. He simply decided to spend his life building bridges, trying to fix what is broken in our society. He visited soup kitchens and hospitals. He supported the Make-A-Wish Foundation, the Special Olympics, and summer camp for children infected with AIDS. There is no shortage of good work in his bio and more than anything his life ended with a lesson for us all in tolerance and understanding and the idea that heroes are human.

In only one lifetime, he went from being hated to being adored. He is the epitome of what is possible if we dare to courageously open our hearts and minds. Somehow an airport bearing his name helps remind us all of the potential… potential to fly… even if you start right here where you are, in Louisville, Kentucky, home of The Greatest of All Time.

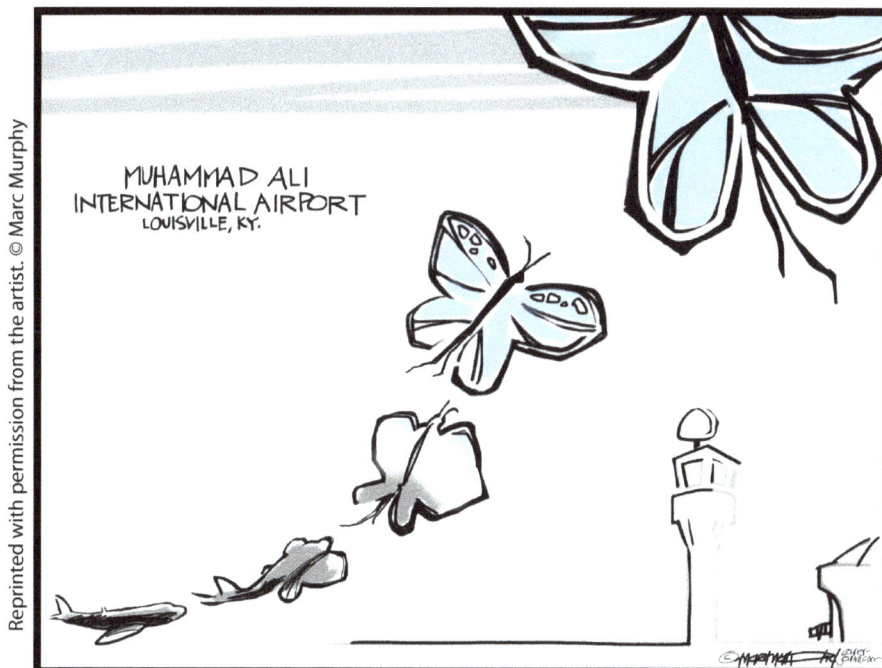

Reprinted with permission from the artist. © Marc Murphy

MUHAMMAD ALI INTERNATIONAL AIRPORT
LOUISVILLE, KY.

STRUCTURAL INEQUALITY, TRANSDISCIPLINARY RESEARCH, AND COMMUNITY EMPOWERMENT

Cedric Merlin Powell, Professor of Law
and Interim Associate Dean for Academic Affairs
University of Louisville Brandeis School of Law

Disproportionate impact is a hallmark of structural inequality, and it is felt across the African American community. It is manifested in the school-to-prison pipeline, environmental racism and its crippling effects on poor neighborhoods, current disheartening trends such as the resurgence of white supremacist hate groups, and social justice issues that impact west Louisville like food deserts, lack of access to quality health care, and exclusion.

To address the systemic problems of structural exclusion and inequality, a group of more than 45 University of Louisville faculty collaborated to form the Co-operative Consortium for Transdisciplinary Social Justice Research (CCTSJR). This approach is much broader than an interdisciplinary approach to scholarship and action; transdisciplinarity is an integrated approach that bridges across disciplines and incorporates scholars, community leaders and activists, students, and even local government in a co-operative committed to inclusion. Advancing

social justice on multiple levels, the CCTSJR seeks to promote the eradication of the present-day effects of past discrimination; to break down barriers of exclusion and ensure that communities of color have access to societal and economic resources like housing, education, and healthcare; and to conceptualize ways to engage and disrupt systemic inequality.

What is unique, innovative, and powerful about the CCTSJR is its intentional commitment to advance research and action to eradicate systems of power that reinforce inequality. This faculty-led and community-driven initiative promises to introduce tangible solutions to address the societal manifestations of structural inequality in Louisville. All of the projects of the CCTSJR are local partnerships with community stakeholders. This is a defining feature of the co-operative consortium projects because community-engaged scholarship is designed to address local problems on the ground.

There are Faculty Research Fellows, who lead teams comprised of faculty members, graduate and undergraduate student researchers, community organizations, and stakeholders. The engagement of these teams is focused on breaking down barriers of exclusion in society. For example, one research team, in partnership with Park Du Valle Community Health Center, is researching the experiential component of treatment for west Louisville residents. This vital information will aid the clinic in making assessments about wellbeing and coping strategies for its

patients. In a community with a median income of $21,733,[55] well-being may be a challenge, and this study will explore how residents experience and express well-being in their communities. This virtually unexplored aspect of the lives of African Americans in west Louisville is intended to critically assess well-being in economically disadvantaged communities, and to reduce health and well-being disparities.

The "Microaggressions in Clinical Medicine" research team, in partnership with the Kentucky

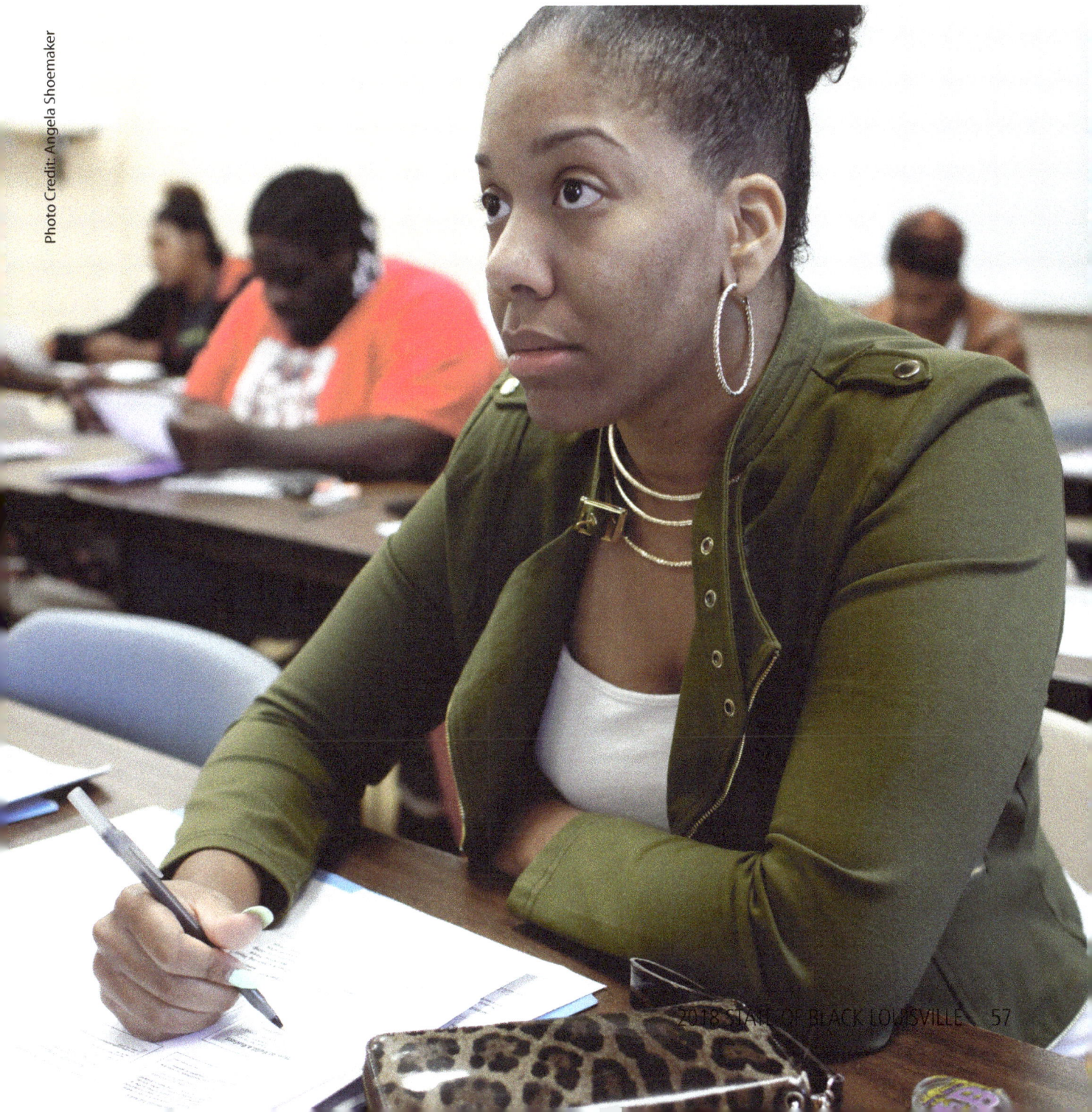

Health Justice Network, is examining the effects of microaggressions – those implicit forms of discriminatory conduct that are ostensibly neutral but devastatingly racist in impact – in clinical medicine and how to avoid them. Professor Peggy Davis further defines microaggressions as "stunning, automatic acts of disregard that stem from unconscious attitudes of white superiority and constitute a verification of black inferiority."[56] Thus, an interaction between a physician and a patient, who is a person of color, could have devastating implications for diagnosis and treatment if the medical professional engages in actions that reinforce feelings of marginalization and inferiority.

This project is designed to identify where those interactions might occur, and provide a critical assessment as to how microaggressions can be avoided. The ultimate goal of the research would be to incorporate this research into the medical school curriculum so that medical professionals will possess a high level of cultural literacy and competency in dealing with diverse patient communities. This project has real implications for west Louisville residents who may be the targets of microaggressions. For example, the research team, in partnership with University of Louisville Pediatrics, with its significant west Louisville patient base, is also focused on offering concrete guidelines to health care providers so that they can avoid committing microaggressions, and eliminate the cyclical effects of toxic stress that disproportionately impact African Americans in west Louisville. This is a critical healthcare access issue.

Community empowerment is essential in dismantling discrimination and societal exclusion, and the "Learning how the Community Leads" research team is critically assessing what it means for west Louisville residents to engage with Louisville Metro-based participatory projects. These participatory projects are unique collaborations between communities and governmental entities that attempt to address specific community challenges. By examining

the processes and collaborations between community and government, the researchers will create responsive tools that enhance community engagement and the policies that are adopted to support these communities.

The segregated housing patterns below the Ninth and Broadway line has long been a historical marker of the centuries-old impact of a state-imposed, residential color line. west Louisville is 81.6% African American.[57] Integrated communities best reflect the societal ideal of inclusion; moreover, fully inclusive communities have better societal resources in terms of jobs, educational opportunities, health and nutrition, and overall quality of life. American life remains largely segregated, and Louisville is no exception. The "Housing Justice in Louisville Metro and Beyond" research team, partnering with the Metropolitan Housing Coalition ("MHC"), will produce an annual state of Metro Louisville housing report, which will be used to develop policies to improve access to housing in integrated communities.

While much progress has been made, we are in a period of retrenchment in which the interests of African Americans, communities of color, and other historically-oppressed groups are largely ignored or viewed as a threat to America's "greatness." We must stand against this cynically-constructed nationalism. These transdisciplinary initiatives will help us to move toward social and economic equality in west Louisville and beyond.

JUDGE HAS DUTY TO DISMISS JURY LACKING DIVERSITY

Sadiqa N. Reynolds, Esq., President and CEO
Louisville Urban League

People of color are still striving for justice in this country, and especially justice in the space where it is supposed to be guaranteed to us all – the courthouse. Does a judge have a right to dismiss a jury panel for lack of diversity? That was the question being debated between Judge Olu Stevens and the Commonwealth's Attorney Tom Wine.

The question went before the Kentucky Supreme Court[58] and the answer to that question, in my opinion, should have been yes. We do not live in a post-racial America, and issues of race and racism exist and hit many of us in the face each and every day. Thus, I would argue that not only does a judge have a right to dismiss a jury for lack of diversity; in fact, he/she ought to have a duty.

I am a lawyer and I know that the law of Batson v. Kentucky is well established. Because of it, courts aren't required to include members of a defendant's race to create a jury of peers. I also am fully aware

that the court had to rule on Batson in 1986 to stop the overt racial profiling that was happening in courtrooms every day. So those that would argue that justice is color blind need only look to the 1986 U.S. Supreme Court ruling in Batson to quickly end that debate.

You are either for continued celebration and honor of those who fought and died, or were willing to die, for the right to systematically subjugate, brutalize and murder an entire race of people based solely on their skin color and desire for wealth or you are not.

The Sixth Amendment to the U.S. Constitution guarantees the accused the right to an impartial jury. If we are to create an impartial jury or even the appearance of one, shouldn't we insist that the jury panel reflects the makeup of the community? Let's review the evidence African Americans have to simply trust the system. Have we not shined enough light on the criminal justice system to prove that it is broken? Haven't we seen hundreds of citizens released from death row and thousands wrongfully convicted?

We should not protect the right to do wrong.

So, as I understand it, the Commonwealth is asking the Kentucky Supreme Court to decide if a judge has the right to dismiss a jury panel for lack of minorities. It is a fair question and I do not believe our Commonwealth's Attorney is endorsing anyone's right to an all-white jury. However, I do understand that if he wins his argument, that could be the effect. I've known both these men for years and think

favorably of both. The issue here is the judge's right to exercise discretion in jury selection – discretion that historically has been very broad.

I refuse to argue about whether or not Judge Stevens violated the law. It's not my point. After all, judges and lawyers make reversible errors every day. That is why we have appellate courts. I'm simply saying if the Kentucky Supreme Court rules that Judge Stevens did violate the law, then the law should be changed and if, in fact, there is no clear case law on the matter, it is past the time for creating it.

Justice is not blind and neither is faith.

Photo: © Meinzahn | Dreamstime.com

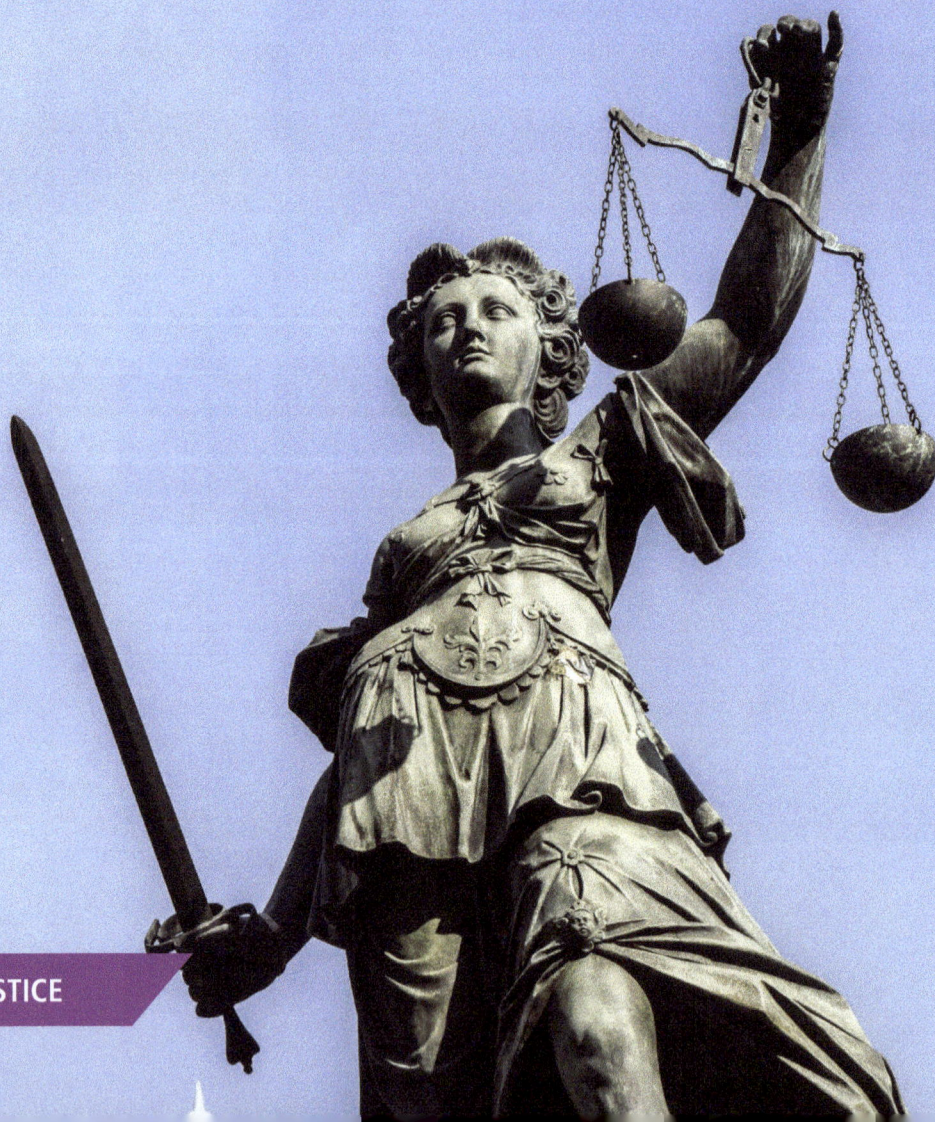

SHIFTING PHILANTHROPY FROM CHARITY TO JUSTICE

Dorian O. Burton, Assistant Executive Director & Chief Program Officer; Co-founder
William R. Kenan, Jr. Charitable Trust
TandemED
Brian C.B. Barnes, Chief Community Officer, Co-founder
Tennessee Achievement School District
TandemED

We need a new framework for giving to address America's economic, social, and political inequalities.

Historical injustices – perpetuated by racial and cultural conflicts and exacerbated by a lack of empathy – are at the heart of America's growing economic, social, and political inequalities. Nowhere is this gap of authentic empathy and justice more pronounced than in the American philanthropic sector, where often well-intentioned people make decisions for communities they do not come from, may not understand, rarely interact with, and almost never step foot into.

"Philanthropy is commendable," said Dr. Martin Luther King, Jr., "but it must not cause the philanthropist to overlook the circumstances of economic injustice, which make philanthropy necessary."[59] Philanthropists and philanthropic advisors who champion equality must work to shift from a framework that grounds giving in "charity" to one that grounds giving in "justice." A framework rooted in charity alone ignores past realities that forced communities into oppressive situations, and risks reinforcing givers' lack of understanding with rewards that recognize their benevolence.

In proposing this fundamental shift, the field should seek to reclaim charitable giving by supporting practices that liberate – and that change the attitudes, beliefs, and policies of – society as a whole. It should seek to break down longstanding, intentional, institutional policies[60] that have shaped social divides in the United States and that continue to promote inequality today.

How can we make this shift? To start, grantmakers and advisors must analyze both the inputs and

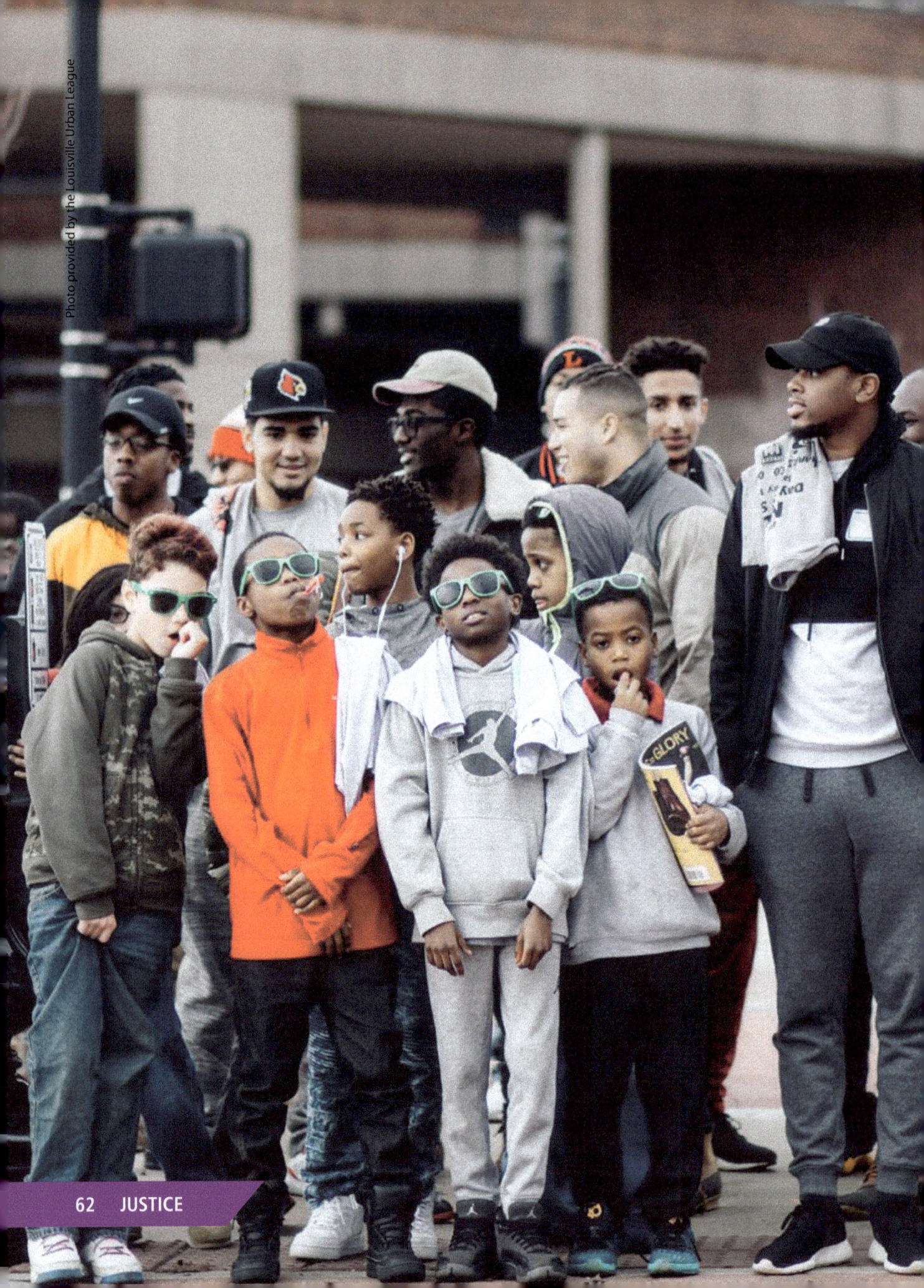

outputs of their philanthropic efforts, with the goal of justice in mind. In doing this, we cannot overstress the importance of beginning with the right set of questions.

Here are seven questions that every philanthropist should consider in their analysis:

ARE YOU AWARE OF AND DO YOU VALUE THE EXISTING LEADERSHIP IN THE COMMUNITY YOU PLAN TO SERVE?

We should begin every initiative with the assumption that there is competent leadership within the communities we aim to serve – people already on the ground, building and changing lives. While some may be under-resourced or untapped, leaders exist in every community. Understand that leadership might look different than what you expect. Seek out people who have a propensity to inspire others to become leaders and who can move a group toward a common goal. These individuals understand the mindsets, perspectives, challenges, opportunities, and attitudes of the community, and unless you spend time with them, you will not see the same assets they see, nor will you be able to truly support the transformation of the community through your collaborative efforts.

Ask: Are we publicly promoting narratives that affirm the leadership of the community? Have we checked our assumptions about whom we deem a leader? Is our organization supportive of the community's leadership strategies?

DO YOU SEE AND UNDERSTAND THE HISTORICAL FACTORS THAT UNDERLIE THE ISSUES YOU AIM TO TACKLE?

Justice-based giving is an act of righting a wrong, leveling the playing field, and removing the illusion of recipients as "less fortunate." It fully acknowledges past the economic, social, and racial disparities that have driven inequalities, and prompts givers to recognize the advantages some groups and individuals have gained over others from years of such injustices.

In his book *The Souls of Black Folks*, W.E.B. Du Bois asks, "How does it feel to be a problem?" The popular "problem-based" narratives ascribed to communities of color are inaccurate and counterproductive. Philanthropic strategies must drop the "problem" tag. One core issue we can correct by using a justice-based framework is the current tendency to set up "funding games," where grantees are pitted against each other, vying to tell the best, most compelling problem-based story about the communities they aim to serve. In this *Mad Max* «thunderdome-style" of grantmaking, philanthropic dollars too often flow to whichever organizations give the best deficit-based narratives – and the worst statistical analyses as to why marginalized communities are poor, disenfranchised, broken, and in need of being "saved" by a targeted intervention. As philanthropists, we must see that we are incentivizing and prolonging myths that continue to oppress those we aim to help.

Ask: Do we support organizations whose mission and vision are built on perpetuating and supporting problem- or deficit-based narratives? If so, how can we help them pivot to build and implement strategies for change rooted in justice?

WHAT IS THE VALUE IN GETTING PROXIMATE TO THOSE YOU SERVE?

Philanthropic organizations must move past the zero-contact grant application process and the feel-good stories of "giving without seeing" often told at homogenous cocktail hours, and strive to get to their boots on the ground, where they can clearly identify how current systems – and in some cases their own practices – are perpetuating injustices.

This kind of *in-person* knowing is what lawyer and social justice activist Bryan Stevenson refers to as "getting proximate to the people you aim to serve."[61] In this proximate stance, we can understand that we are not dealing with people who are inherently challenged or responsible for their own poverty.

Instead, we must acknowledge advantages, privileges, and power dynamics, and approach our work *alongside* individuals to fix or replace broken systems. Engage in meaningful dialogue and develop public kinship. Get out in the community; don't hide or shelter yourself from the people you are charged with serving.

Ask: Is getting proximate to the community you serve – to listen, learn, and partner – core to your organization's theory of change or action? Does every individual at your organization, including the board chair and the office coordinator, have an intimate understanding and knowledge of the communities they are tasked with serving?

DO YOU SEE GRANTEES AND COMMUNITY LEADERS AS EQUAL PARTNERS IN YOUR PHILANTHROPIC STRATEGY?

It's important not to create power dynamics by placing your own organization at the top of a hierarchy. Be on tap, not on top. We must rework or remove common practices such as investing in already-envisioned initiatives or holding listening sessions that have no impact on how a social effort moves forward. These practices use the community as a type of insurance policy for buy-in, rather than as a partner who has the competence to meaningfully contribute. True community engagement requires that all parties listen with an empathetic ear, contribute ideas and perspectives, and then wrap whatever expertise and resources they have around community leaders in an effort to bring their dreams to fruition.

Ask: Are there mindsets and assumptions among the people at your organization that do not cast grantees and the community you serve in an "equal" light? Do you believe you have only something to give, as opposed to something to learn, from those you aim to partner with?

DO YOU SEE THE VALUE OF INCLUDING DIVERSE PERSONS ON YOUR OWN TEAM?

Between 1980 and 2000, the minority population in the United States increased by 88%.[62] Further, racial and ethnic minorities were responsible for 91.7% of U.S. population growth between 2000 and 2010, and although minorities make up about 37% of the U.S. population, 50.4% of the children born in 2011 were part of a racial or ethnic minority.[63]

There are and will continue to be ample opportunities to find people to enhance staff diversity – not only in terms of race and ethnicity, or gender, but also in terms of socioeconomic status and proximity to communities we serve. Increased creativity, satisfaction, productivity, synergy, and wellbeing in the workplace are among the potential positive impacts of diversity.[64] As people with different experiences and approaches to problem solving interact and make connections between previously unrelated agents, goods, and knowledge, innovation tends to increase.

Ask: Do your organizational, executive, and program teams reflect the population of the communities you serve, or are you internally propagating the inequalities your program portfolios are tasked with changing?

DO YOU SEE THE VALUE OF SMALLER ORGANIZATIONS?

It is easy to assume that smaller organizations have less potential for impact than larger ones. But small organizations are often embedded in a community's day-to-day activities. As such, they have deep insight into the community and its history, and, given proper resources (especially long-term general operating support and other flexible resources), a strong ability to propel justice-driven change.

Ask: Does your organization tend to avoid working with smaller organizations on the ground? Are you funding organizations led by individuals who reflect the communities you wish to impact? How might you use your own influence to connect smaller organizations with the goal of increasing opportunities for impact?

IS YOUR ORGANIZATION ACCOUNTABLE TO DRIVING SYSTEMS-LEVEL CHANGE?

Individual communities and philanthropic program efforts often engage in siloed causes that do not necessarily lead to systemic change. In a justice-based framework, all program activities act in a coordinated manner to create a new systems-level "normal" that solidifies justice and dismantles inequalities for the communities we serve. By supporting opportunities for collaboration among grantees, we can tackle adaptive challenges and avoid mission creep. If grantees are creating reports that live and die on our desks, it is a waste of their time and a missed opportunity to bring bright spot models (or examples of excellence) into the national conversation for change. Part of our job as grantmakers is to get the word out, and work with advocacy organizations and policy makers to turn effective programs into sustainable policies.

We must also look at the metrics we are holding our own organizations – not just our grantees – accountable to. Systems of checks and balances that rest solely with the board, or that don't include the community in the governance structure, might be missing the mark. Accountability rooted in community values and vision is also essential—what is good for the gander should also be good for the golden goose.

Ask: Do you support advocacy organizations that help build awareness and civic engagement around justice-oriented, systems-level reforms? Do you give your grantees space and room to work collaboratively with other organizations? How can your network support grantees' efforts in transforming programs into scalable policies beyond local efforts? How is your organization holding itself accountable and to who?

Ultimately, real change will come only when all organizations and individuals in a system change. But systemic change does not come without expense. Time, resources, reputation, and relationships all require adjustments and sacrifice as we move from charitable giving to a justice-based framework of philanthropy. The question becomes: Are we as philanthropists, in the name of justice, willing to pay the cost for the change we wish to see? Our actions moving forward will reveal our answer.

Charity is commendable, but justice is transformational. How will you spend your resources?

"I WRITE ABOUT RACE BECAUSE … WE ARE NOT YOUR SLAVES!"

Dr. Ricky L. Jones, Professor & Chair
Pan-African Studies Department, University of Louisville

To the chagrin of many readers, I often write about race. My harshest critics (and there is certainly a nice little cadre who complain early and often after the publication of almost every column) will be surprised to know that I do not write about race so much because I enjoy it. I would actually like to write more about other things – sports, love, sci-fi, or how I was depressed and angry after seeing the long-awaited, but absolutely terrible cinematic butchering of Stephen King's "The Dark Tower." I do not write about race because I want to; I write about race because I have to.

Situations like what happened in Charlottesville, Virginia tell you why I write about race. Charlottesville is not new – even though the talking heads on television speak as if it is. Contrary to those prone to oversimplify, it is not the result of the Donald Trump phenomenon; he is simply a socio-political conduit. There is no rise in White supremacist sentiment; it has always been there. The "White identitarian" worldview is not limited to "out in the open" nationalists; they are just more upfront about it and in touch with their racism.

I write about race because the subject deserves and demands constant, historically rooted, intelligent engagement. It is an ever-present reality, not something to be shallowly blathered about at disconnected point-instants. It is not a subject for CNN, Fox News, MSNBC, or local news sound bites featuring frustratingly ineffective dilettantes. For them, incidents from Ferguson to Staten Island to New Orleans to Charlottesville are "stories." They will

I write about race because deformed systems create deformed human beings. Our racially diseased national organism bends and breaks people.

move on to the next "hot thing" very quickly. Black people cannot afford to do so. For us, this is life.

I write about race because we must understand connections and the proverbial full picture. Even as we witness the contrived indignation and surprise of many White Americans that the president did not immediately and full-throatedly condemn White supremacists by name after Charlottesville, we understand it is difficult for a man who has brought White supremacists into his White House to do so. We understand a civil rights investigation by a Department of Justice led by the likes of Attorney General Jeff Sessions who is riddled with racial insensitivity is also laughable.

I write about race because most "successful" Blacks who are fiercely committed to being "politically correct" and "playing the game" will not.

I write about race because deformed systems create deformed human beings. Our racially diseased national organism bends and breaks people. To be sure, many blacks do not wish to carry the burden of race and escape into the recesses of their minds. This yields the twisted Jenean Hamptons, Sammy Sosas, Ward Conerlys, O.J. Simpsons, Shelby Steeles, and Omarosa Manigaults of the world. They are sad representations of misguided, vulgar-careerist Black zombies who care more about money, position, and acceptance than they do about preserving the humanity or lives of children.

I write about race because there are people who argue the issue does not exist and those who raise it are the real problem. I write about it because most Black people do not have the access or opportunity to do so. They are silenced in ghettoes, drudgery, struggle, and the numbness of addiction to escape the madness of their worlds. I write about race

because most "successful" Blacks who are fiercely committed to being "politically correct" and "playing the game" will not. They have succumbed to cowardice, ignorance, indifference, and callousness. They will not open their mouths because they are terrified of losing employment, funding, or friendship of Whites who claim to love them ... until they stand up and tell any modicum of truth. They puff and preen because of professional achievements, but are little more than empty shells who contribute nothing to the global humanization project.

I write about race because every generation yields a small number of courageous and credentialed Americans who have dared to do so. From W. E. B Dubois to Ida B. Wells-Barnett to Zora Neale Hurston to Langston Hughes to Audre Lorde, there is a tradition of such writers turning newspapers, magazines, and books into classrooms. They have taught, challenged, and changed. These giants provide a standard writers like myself will never reach, but must always aspire. They scream from the grave that we cannot allow ourselves to become hollowed- out husks, nauseatingly preoccupied with making critics comfortable and paralyzed by equivocation.

I write about race because we always need Black intellectuals who stand and scream, "We are not your slaves! We are not your cowards! We are not your co-signers! Harkening back to James Baldwin, we are not your negroes!" Some of us must extend ourselves. We must expose our tender parts to the mob and take their blows. We must risk. And yes, some of us must suffer and die. But that paves the way for others to be braver, more enlightened, and more human.

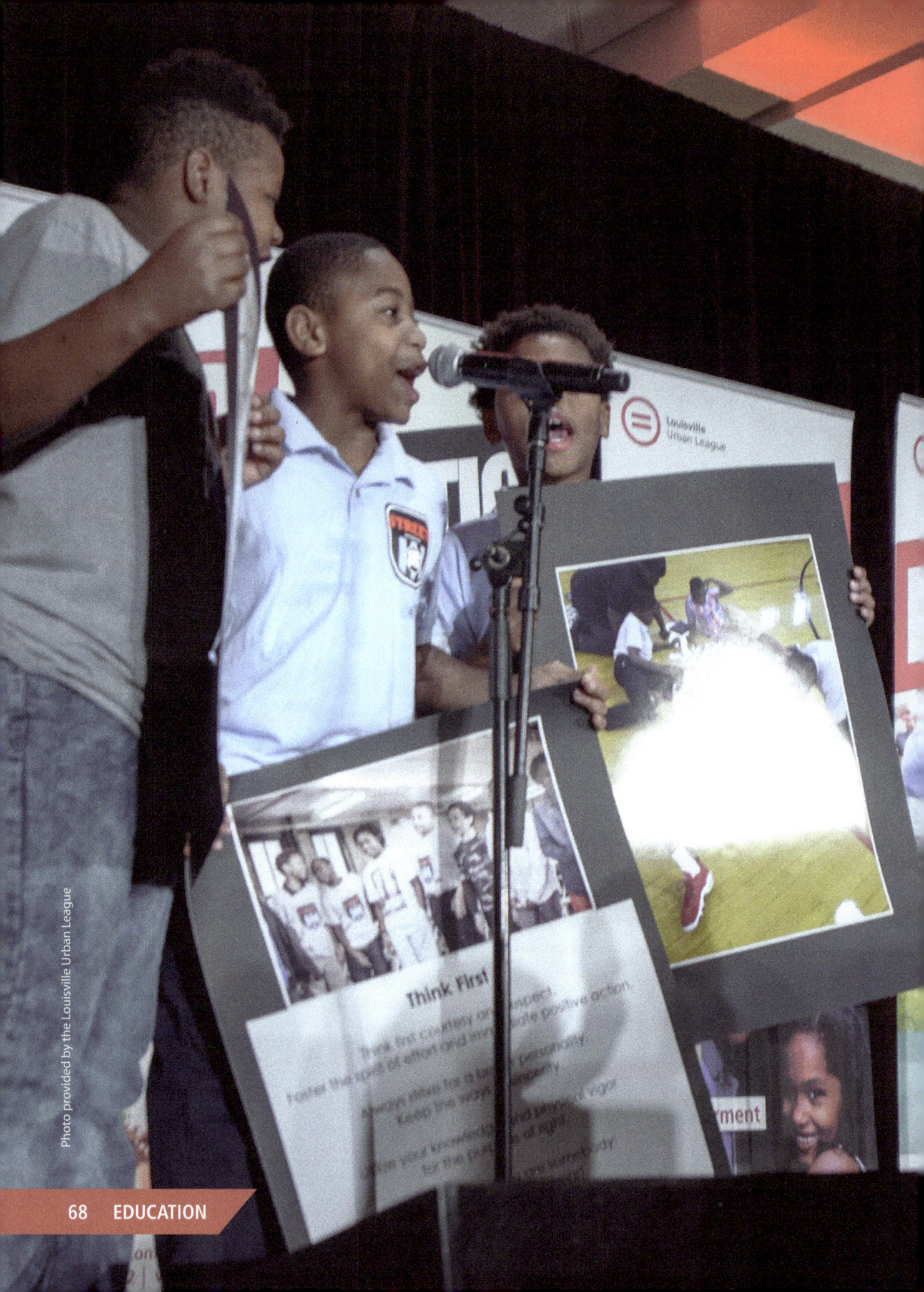

EDUCATION
AND YOUTH DEVELOPMENT

The largest school district in the state is the Jefferson County Public School (JCPS) system, which enrolls 99,910, students.[65] The largest city in the state, Louisville, is a part of the JCPS system and nearly half of all African American public school students in Kentucky attend schools in Jefferson County.[66]

We must work to close achievement gaps and promote equal education for all by strengthening our communities so that our children have safe, enriching environments in which they can learn and develop, and where good grades are the expectation and not the exception. Among other education issues in Louisville, we should be concerned about:

▶ Increasing the number of Black teachers. In the 1953-54 school year (64 years ago), 6.8% of our state's teachers were African American. The percentage has dropped below 3%. In JCPS, African American students are 37% of the student population. However, African American teachers are only 3.5% of teachers in the county.[67] [68]

▶ School board composition. When we look at the racial breakdown of school board members in Kentucky, we see that, according to reports from the Kentucky Department of Education, there are 667 White members and only 37 non-White members. In Louisville, there is only one African American member of the school board.[69]

▶ School-to-prison pipeline. Disproportionate suspension rates, push-out rates, zero tolerance policies, and other discipline issues contribute directly to increased dropout rates and school-to-prison pipelines. In Jefferson County during the 2016- 2017 school year, out of 8,845 high school students suspended, 5,652 were African American.[70]

State and city plans related to education are currently being made. Some plans could lead public school districts toward equity and opportunity. Other plans could lead us down a path to privatization and disinvestment. We must make sure that the African American community has a seat at the table as these plans are being discussed. Issues related to school choice, vouchers, charter schools, private schools, etc., all require additional studies and expanded community dialogue.

We must not allow our educational institutions to drift back toward racially-segregated systems. Our children's lives matter. We must ensure that every child has access to and obtains a meaningful and first-rate education.

John J. Johnson, Executive Director
Kentucky Commission on Human Rights

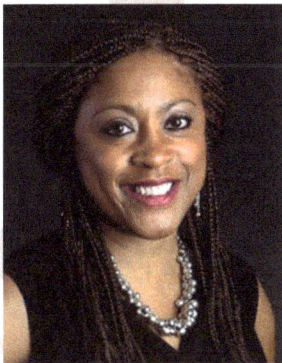

DANA JACKSON, Better Together Strategies, LLC

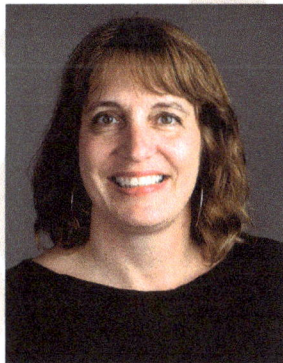

JENNIE JEAN DAVIDSON, Better Together Strategies, LLC

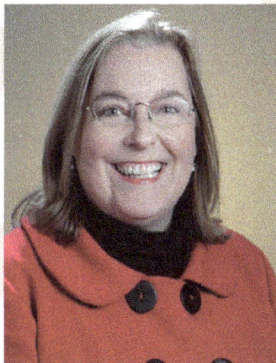

DR. ANITA P. BARBEE, University of Louisville

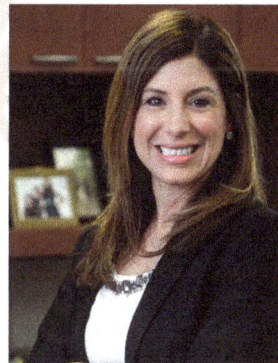

THERESA RENO-WEBER, Metro United Way

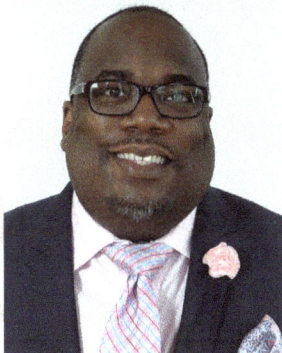

DARYLE UNSELD, JR., Metro United Way

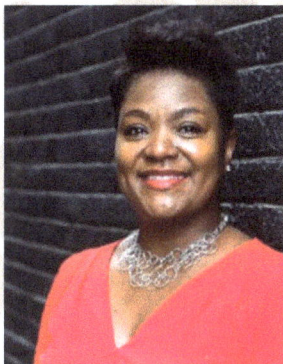

SADIQA N. REYNOLDS, ESQ., Louisville Urban League

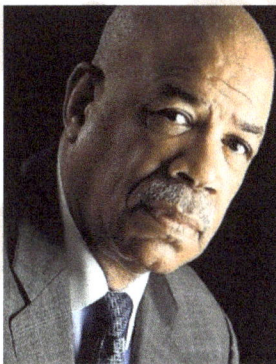

RAOUL CUNNINGHAM, Louisville Branch of the NAACP

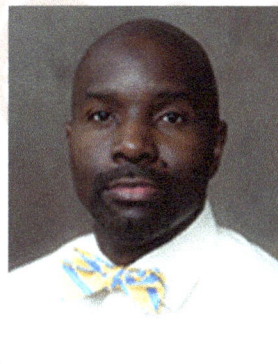

DR. AHMAD WASHINGTON, University of Louisville

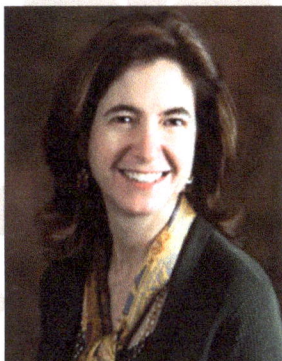

MARY GWEN WHEELER, 55,000 Degrees

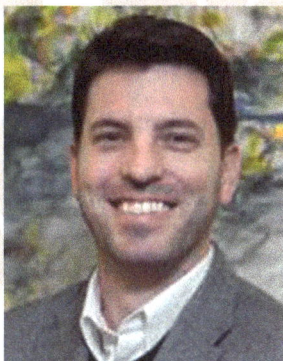

DR. MATT BERRY, 55,000 Degrees

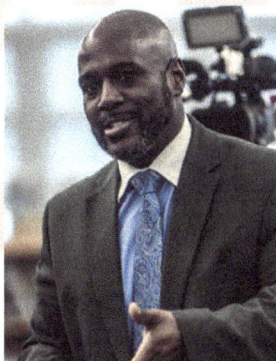

DR. JOHN MARSHALL, Jefferson County Public Schools

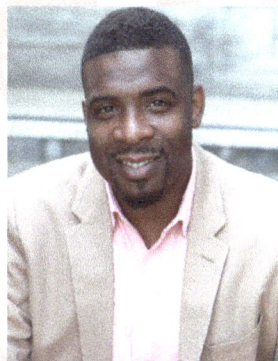

TIMOTHY E. FINDLEY, JR., Kingdom Fellowship Christian Life Center

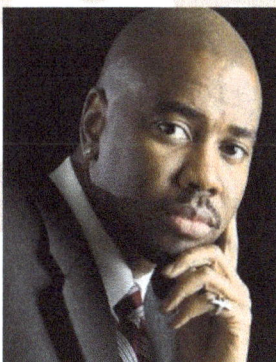

DR. RICKY L. JONES, University of Louisville

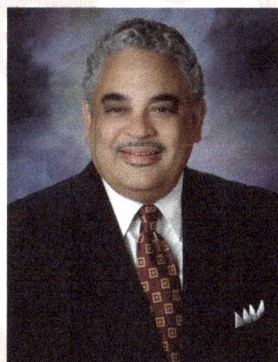

JOHN J. JOHNSON, Kentucky Commission on Human Rights

STANDING IN THE GAP: 15,000 DEGREES ADDRESSES THE OPPORTUNITY GAP

Dana Jackson, Consultant

Jennie Jean Davidson, Consultant

Better Together Strategies, LLC

Better Together Strategies, LLC is a consultant for the 15K Degrees Initiative.

The racial achievement gap is dangerous and persistent. It oozes into every corner of education, from early years through college graduation. Unequal outcomes limit African American students' futures and the fundamental promise of education – a path toward economic prosperity.

For years, the education discourse has focused on the achievement gap. Finally, however, the work to close this breach is shifting to focus on the "opportunity gap." Think of the gap this way: the opportunity gap is the *cause* and the achievement gap is the *effect*. The opportunity gap shows up when families can't afford excellent preschool, when kids can't learn because they go to school hungry, when "certain" schools are under resourced, when college is too costly. Addressing it requires a commitment to excellence in education for each, every, and all students. It requires educators, advocates, and community to look at all the ways that race, ethnicity, socio-economic status, community wealth (or lack thereof), and other factors contribute to lower educational aspirations, achievement, and attainment. [71]

The work is urgent; there is much to do. Starting in kindergarten, Jefferson County's African American students are less ready than their White schoolmates (43% vs 55%), creating a steep climb from the start. The gap persists: in elementary school, only 29% of Black students score at "proficient or above" compared to 58% of White students. Too few students take Advanced Placement exams in high school. Last year only 18% of those students were African American.

Later measures paint a sobering picture: only 44.7% of African American students graduate ready for college or career – a picture of limited opportunities

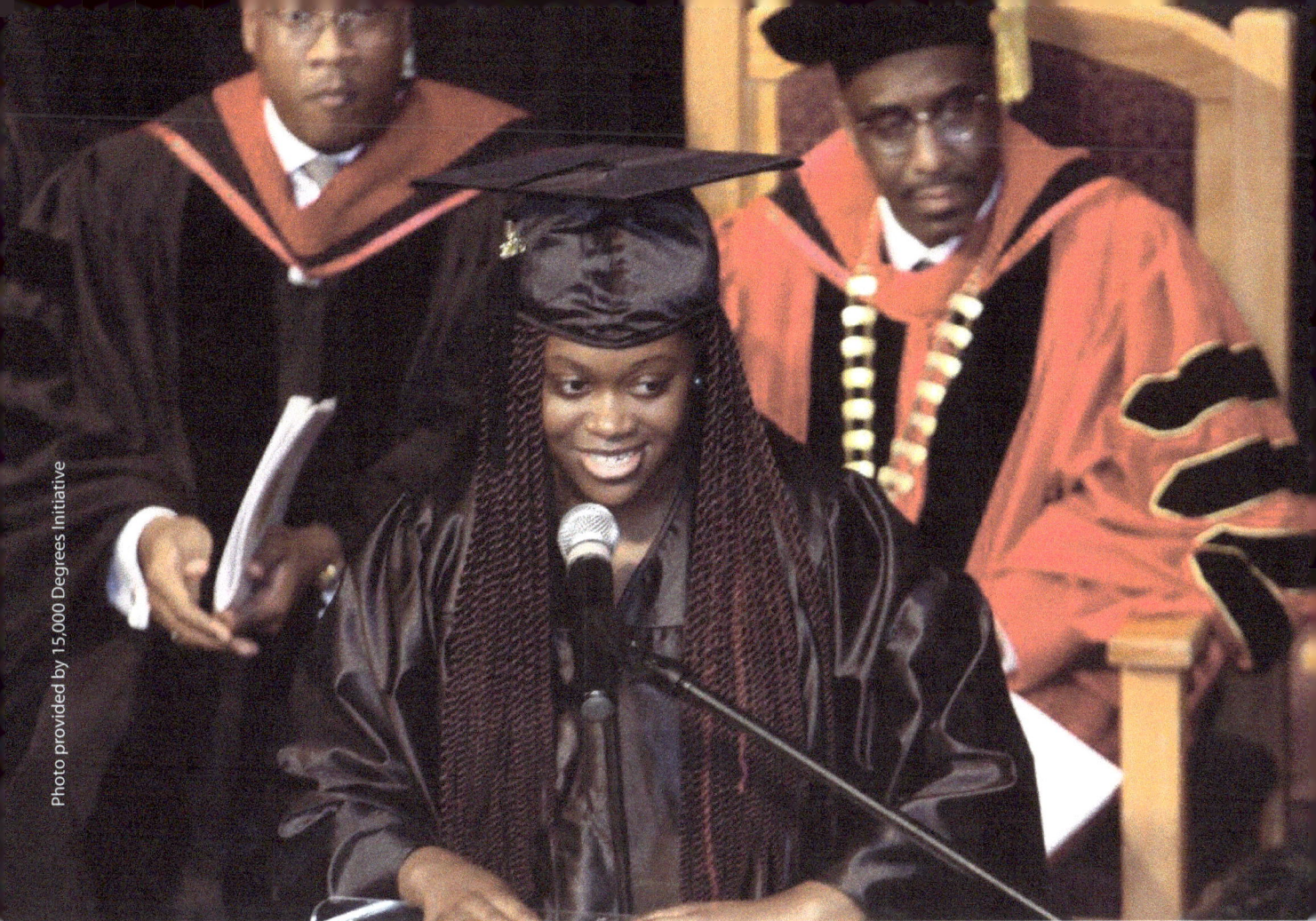

and a system that is not preparing students for college.[72] The gap also shows up in college completion. Of nearly 9,000 two- and four-year degrees conferred by area colleges and universities in 2016, only 12% were earned by African Americans.[73]

Why do these measures matter? Kindergarten readiness sets children up for a strong start. Reading proficiency is a crucial marker: until 3rd grade, students *learn to read* and for the rest of their educational career they *read to learn*. Advanced Placement classes give students an important head start in college. And the numbers on the value of a post-secondary degree are clear: average weekly earnings are 40% higher for a college graduate.[74]

Equitable, excellent education is not just the job of the schools. To disrupt these pervasive negative outcomes, our community must work at a scale that makes a significant difference, not just for a few of our students, but for all. There is no one solution. It will take a multi-faceted approach across the education continuum.

15,000 Degrees is committed to increasing the number of African American degrees by 15,000 by 2020. We engage and mobilize the Louisville African American community in support of enhanced education attainment, support systems that yield more equitable education outcomes and access, and seek to ignite a community vision that advances college readiness and accelerates a culture of college-going and degree completion.

RECOMMENDATIONS

▶ **Address the Opportunity Gap.**
Make equity the foundation of our education system. Our school system is doing important work on equity and needs your voice,

presence, and push to work toward equitable outcomes. Attend JCPS School Board meetings and get to know your School Board representative. Ask questions about positions on equity and achievement. Don't know who represents you on the School Board? Start here: *https://www.jefferson.kyschools.us/about/leadership/board-education*

► **Think Bigger.**
We must expand our definition of "education interventions." Housing, public transportation, safety, mental health, health care, and jobs are education interventions. Students can't learn when they are hungry, homeless, scared, or struggling with mental health issues. Families can't engage when constantly worried about joblessness, insufficient wages, health, and safety. We have strong partnerships that work across sectors with the common aim to close the opportunity gap, and they need our support to do more. The Louisville Urban League is a sterling example of a nonprofit that partners for change. Get connected to nonprofits in our community and support them with your time, with your voice, and with financial contributions that allow them to continue doing their important work.

► **Change the System**.
Programs and services are important responses to the very real challenges students and families experience, but they alone are insufficient to achieve the change we need. System change will be required to disrupt the racialized outcomes we see – low achievement, low college-going, and graduation. Without attention to policy, "the fix" is applied only to students and families and not to the broken parts of the system that churn out uneven outcomes. Learn about the policies and laws that govern our school system and post-secondary institutions and understand their impact,

particularly on racial equity and educational attainment. Learn about your elected officials. Run for office yourself!

► **Get Active.**
Shine a light on bias and strategies for addressing it. Use data to illuminate inequitable outcomes. Unapologetically, point out and provide feedback on statements and actions that perpetuate bias and uneven outcomes for African American students.   Join policy-making bodies and boards that focus on education, social supports, and civil rights. Show up and voice concerns at school board meetings. Support efforts, like 15,000 Degrees, that remove barriers to college access, affordability, and graduation. Look for evidence-based practices that are working, here and elsewhere.

► **Stand in the Gap**.
Use your networks, power, and voice to address the opportunity gap. Be a bridge to better outcomes by giving of yourself with your time, talent, and treasure. Volunteer in the schools. Connect with students and families to hear what's working and what's not. Speak up for our students and families. Our students need us.

THE CHILD WELFARE SYSTEM IN BLACK LOUISVILLE

Dr. Anita P. Barbee, Professor

Kent School of Social Work, University of Louisville

The child welfare system was developed in order to ensure child safety. In Kentucky and in Louisville, the child welfare system is housed within the Department for Community Based Services (DCBS) in the Permanency and Protection unit. There, workers receive calls regarding any suspected child abuse, neglect, or abandonment. These allegations of maltreatment are thoroughly investigated and if maltreatment is substantiated, then the case is opened. Sometimes, the children remain in the home and other times children are removed from the home to kinship or foster care while the caseworker helps the family make changes needed to improve child safety.

The goal is to move as quickly as possible to achieve child safety and reunify families before closing the case. In those instances where insufficient progress is made towards ensuring the child can safely remain in or return to the home or the home of extended family, then there is a move to have the child(ren) adopted so that the child can grow up in a permanent, loving family.

Kentucky has a particularly overburdened system since our child poverty rates are high and our child maltreatment rates (20.6 per 1,000) are more than double the national average (9.4 per 1,000).[75] As a result, the outcomes of safety, permanency, and well-being for families and children who encounter our system are not always met. This is particularly true for African American families where great disproportionality and disparities exist. In Louisville, African American children are disproportionally removed from their homes into the foster care system at a rate one and a half times that of White children.[76] And once they are in foster care, African American children and their families receive fewer services and the children are disproportionally less likely to return to parent or a kin provider or become adopted.

More African American children end up leaving the

foster care system at age 18 without a family to rely on during the precarious transition to the early adult years.[77]

In July 2017, a *New York Times* article referred to the way the child welfare system interacts with African American families as the new "Jane Crow", meaning poor African American and Hispanic mothers are held to higher standards than other parents.[78] It also stated that some removals are meant to "punish parents with few resources…", which is essentially the "criminalization of their parenting choices." Removal of children from their family is traumatizing to the children and is devastating to parents.

There are several potential solutions to this problem.

RAISE AWARENESS AND MOBILIZATION.

The Race Community and Child Welfare (RCCW) Committee has been in existence for 12 years to address this issue. Between 2005 and 2008, over 1,000 professionals within DCBS, the courts, and the school, mental health, and health systems were trained by the People's Institute for Survival and Beyond in *Undoing Racism*. This is a two-day workshop constructed to raise awareness of what racism is, where it comes from, how it functions, why it persists, and how it can be undone. When the impact of the training was evaluated, it was found that participants significantly gained knowledge and improved in anti-racism attitudes. Follow-up surveys found that participants were mobilized to give presentations about diversity and *Undoing Racism* at work, made policy and practice changes, and engaged in case reviews to prevent discrimination. The positive impact of the training lasted up to four years and disparities in the child welfare system improved for a time.[79] [80]

Unfortunately, the funding was cut and the training ended. With renewed interest by DCBS, the RCCW group has developed a new day-long training session that is ready for dissemination to professionals in child welfare agencies, the courts, schools, and healthcare. Hopefully this success story can once again stem the tide of disproportionate outcomes for

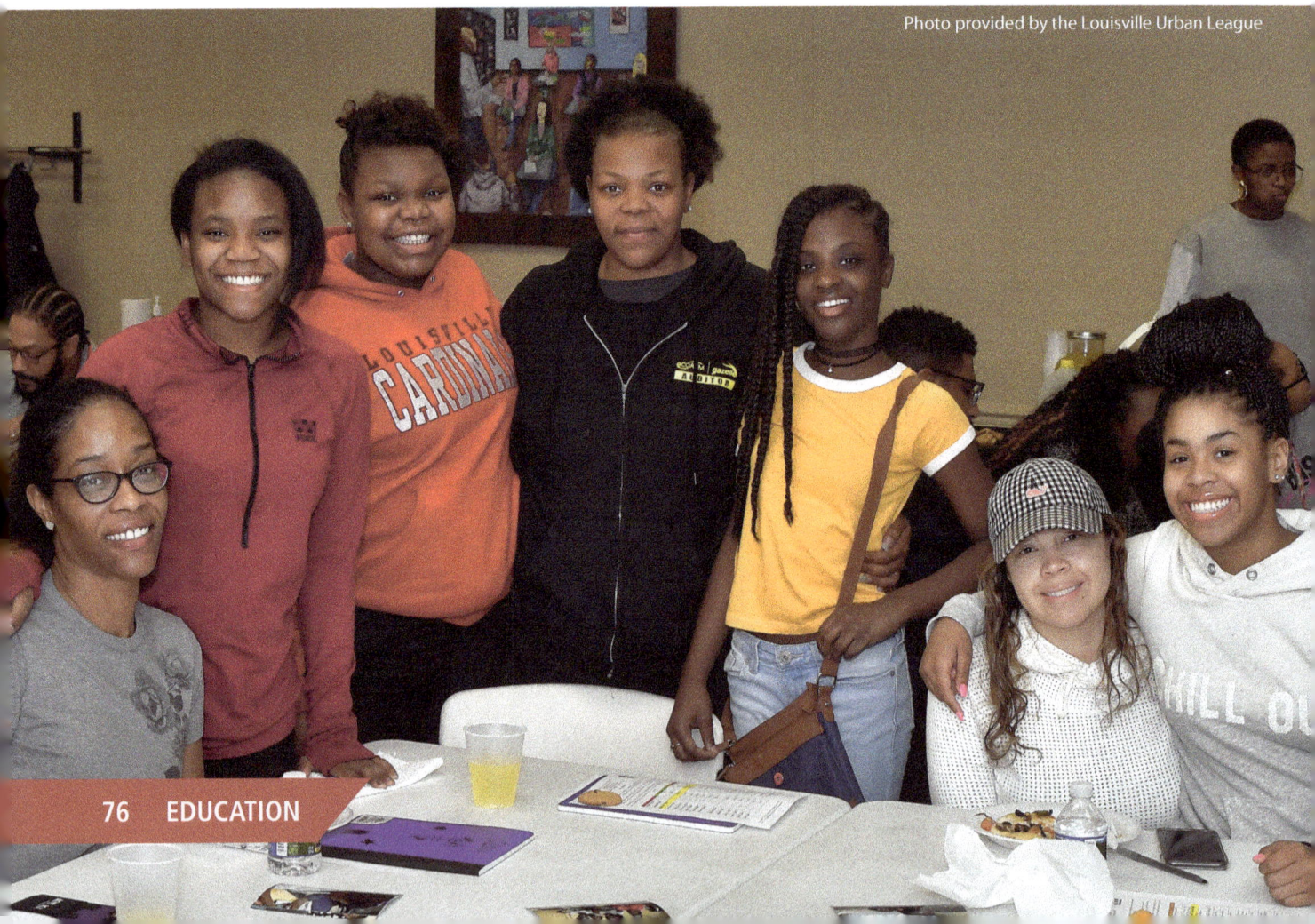

Photo provided by the Louisville Urban League

African American children in the child welfare system.

But, it is not enough to simply change the child welfare system directly. Circumstances that undermine the Black family must also be addressed.

TARGET EFFORTS AT REDUCING POVERTY AND ITS CONCENTRATION.

Much of the problem involves the disproportionate impoverishment of Black families. There are several systemic strategies to help lift Black families out of poverty including:

► Improving schools so that youth receive the fundamentals essential to succeed in a job, an entrepreneurial venture, or college

► Stopping the practice of concentrating poverty, especially among African Americans. Several strategies are needed to make this a reality:

a) Ensuring that there is enough safe, low-income housing for families all over the community

b) Fighting redlining: the practice of denying services, directly or through raising prices to residents of certain areas – like West Louisville – based on the racial or ethnic composition of those areas

► Bringing investment and jobs closer to where African Americans currently live while enhancing transportation to existing jobs

► Changing the criminal justice system to reduce the unnecessary incarceration of a quarter of Black males, many of whom exit prison without additional job skills or the ability to vote and stay engaged in society.[81]

ENHANCE SUPPORT OF BLACK FAMILIES.

Enhance supports for all families, but particularly poor and African American families by:

► Securing additional funding for family home

visiting programs so that all new mothers receive a family visitor during pregnancy and in the first few years of life to enhance attachment and parenting skills. Currently, family home visitor programs operate out of the Louisville Metro Department of Public Health and Wellness through several of the Neighborhood Places (Healthy Start and HANDS).

► Building more natural supports among mothers raising children like the Metro United Way Ages and Stages program, which engages parent navigators to network with families in West Louisville neighborhoods.

► Joining Community Coordinated Child Care (4Cs) in ensuring there is affordable, high-quality child care available so that mothers can work knowing their children are safe and thriving in a regulated child care setting.

► Investing in out-of-school-time organizations, which keep children busy and active before and after school with an emphasis on empowerment, engagement, and enhanced school performance. Examples include the Cabbage Patch Settlement House, St. George Scholar Institute, and the West Louisville Boys and Girls Choirs.

Most Black families in Louisville are thriving and show tremendous resilience in the face of oppression. Many citizens and leaders are committed to reducing poverty while enhancing neighborhoods and programming so that Black families continue their upward trajectory. May these positive forces in our community never give up, but persist even in the face of great opposition!

LIVING UNITED: THE PATH FORWARD

Theresa Reno-Weber, President & CEO
Daryle Unseld Jr., Director of Community Engagement
Metro United Way

For 100 years, Metro United Way (MUW) has been dedicated to improving lives in our community and that will never change. Along with our strong network of community partners, including the Louisville Urban League, which we've worked alongside and supported since 1921, we are committed to reaching our vision that every individual, child, and family achieves their full potential and succeeds in life.

We bring together the people and resources needed to tackle our community's most significant challenges, because we know that no one person or organization can remove all the barriers preventing people from thriving. In Louisville, those barriers disproportionally affect communities of color and we are determined to change that.

In partnership with several national and local organizations, including the Louisville Urban League, Metro United Way has undertaken many new

strategies and initiatives. Working directly with our national partner, the Association of Black Foundation Executives (ABFE), we are developing a deeper focus on responsive grantmaking with an intentional equity lens tailored to support Black male achievement. ABFE's mission is to promote effective and responsive philanthropy in Black communities. We work with ABFE to gain additional knowledge related to reducing gaps in racial disparities in the philanthropic sector and on how to be more responsive to issues of equity, diversity, and inclusion.

In 2017, Metro United Way piloted a new investment process for our out-of-school time (OST) partners – $420,600 invested in 21 newly funded partners – that emphasizes quality program standards and increases access of opportunities for youth being served by organizations led by people of color. The new investment allows a number of smaller organizations the opportunity to gain a formalized funding partnership with MUW that will promote mutual learning and demonstrate their value and efficacy to our community.

Through our Black Male Achievement (BMA) initiative, we understand the necessity to value all people and invest in Black males as assets, and are working to accelerate practices that continue to improve the life outcomes of African American men and boys in our community. Most recently, Metro United Way developed a partnership with BMe Community and introduced the organization to the nonprofit ecosystem in Louisville. BMe Community is an award-winning network that resets expectations on race, community, and America's future by building more caring and prosperous communities inspired by Black men. Together, we believe BMA, MUW, and other local partners can reshape narratives associated with Black men and boys in Louisville through the asset framing concept (utilizing messaging to define people and communities by their authentic contributions, as opposed to their deficits), as well as the investments in Black male social entrepreneurs BMA makes in their partner cities.

We know through our partnership with BMe Community that there are far more Black males in colleges than in prisons[82]; that according to the U.S. Army, Black men serve this country in uniform at a higher rate than all other men[83]; and the rate of business creation by Black males has been growing at nearly twice the national average for more than a decade, according to the U.S. Census[84].

As we move forward on this journey with our

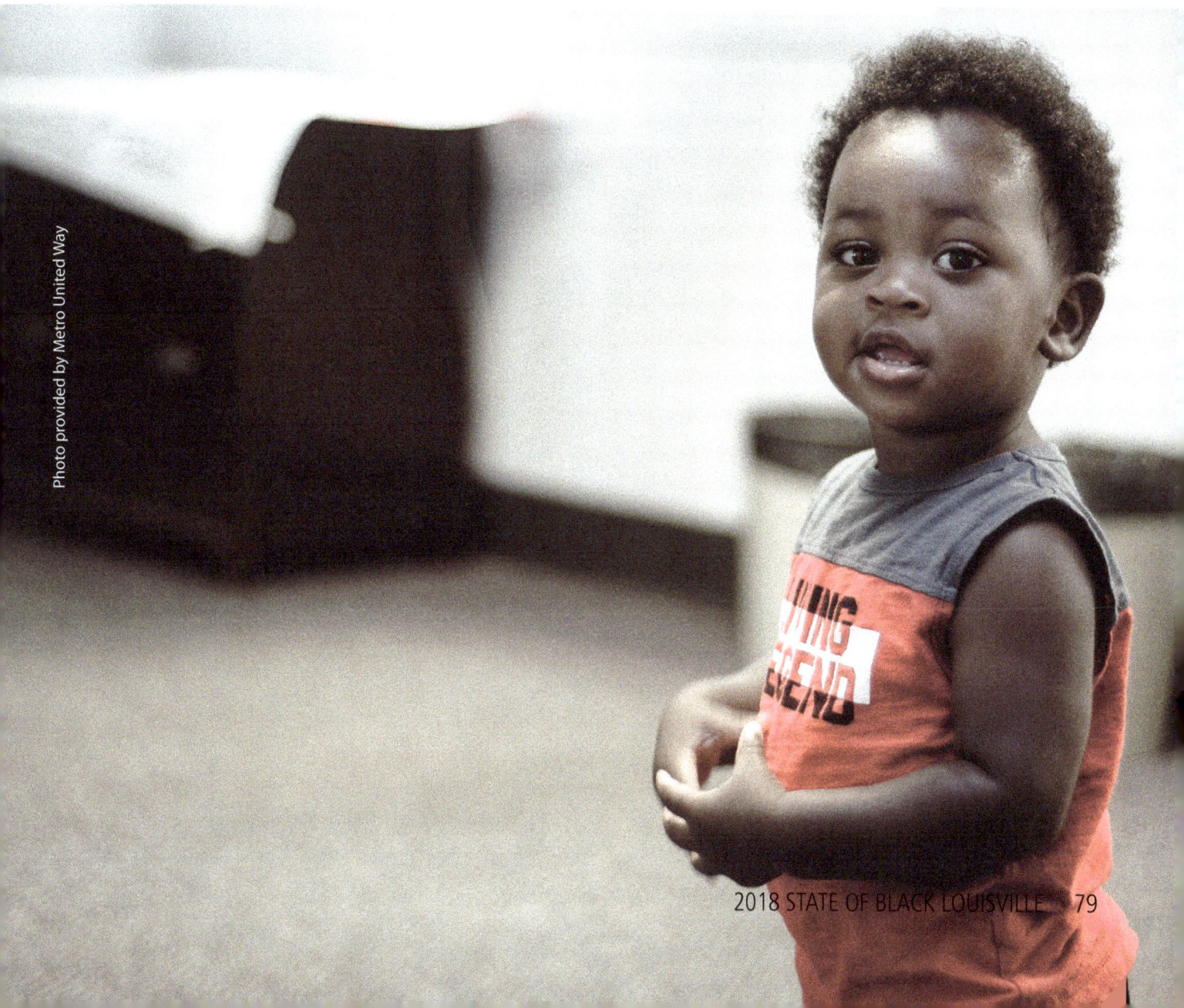

Photo provided by Metro United Way

community, we are committed to the following:

- ▶ Lead with data disaggregated by race and gender to design policies, programs, and grantmaking strategies.

- ▶ Use an intentional racial equity lens to analyze the impact of any proposed policy or programs sponsored by Metro United Way.

- ▶ Message issues facing people and communities responsibly, focused on an asset frame as opposed to deficient messaging.

- ▶ Be deliberate and strategic in the development of culturally-responsive, innovative solutions that work with families and communities to fight for the education, health, and financial independence of all.

Join us as we tackle our community's toughest challenges and help us fight to improve lives, person by person and family by family, because when we Live United, we don't just change the lives of some; we change what is possible for all.

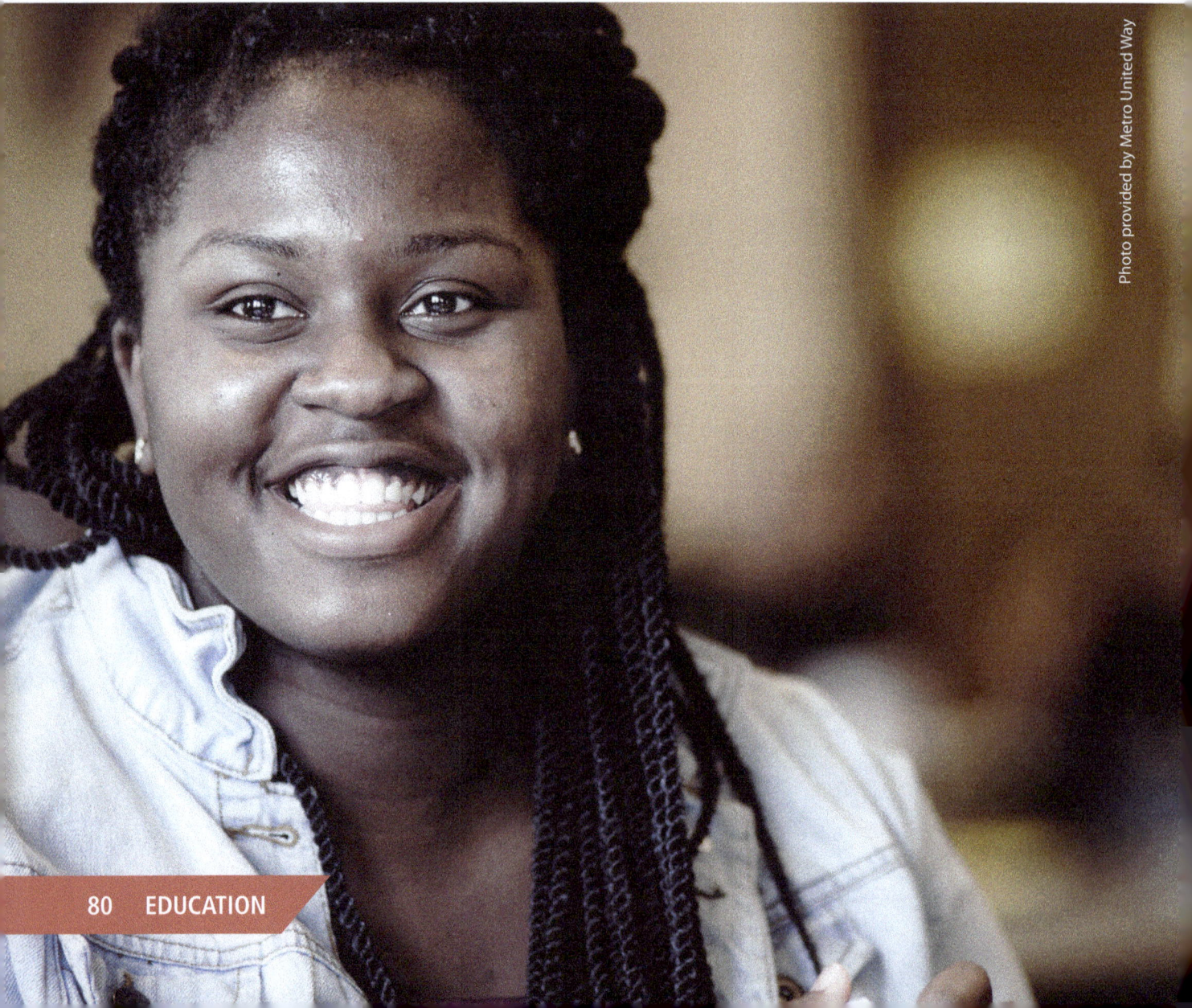

Photo provided by Metro United Way

GOOD ENOUGH NOT GOOD ENOUGH FOR STUDENTS

Sadiqa N. Reynolds, ESQ., President and CEO
Louisville Urban League
Raoul Cunningham, President
Louisville Branch of the NAACP

Kentucky education leaders are now in the process of developing plans to implement a new state education accountability model under the Every Student Succeeds Act (ESSA). The federal law honors citizen engagement in the success of our students and our schools. It is imperative parents, educators, and community members work alongside state officials to ensure all young people, and especially those who have been left behind for too long, have access to a first-rate education.

As citizens, parents, education leaders, and policymakers participate in the process, meaningful systems of accountability are the top priority. We must set high education standards benchmarked to the rigors of college, careers, and civic engagement for all children, including traditionally-disadvantaged student groups. We must set the bar high, knowing students achieve to the expectations we set for them, and communicate clearly what those goals are so that parents can support their children's learning.

In the same way, high-quality assessments and clear reporting are critical because they inform teachers and parents what's working, what's not, and how they can make improvements. We must write down and say out loud what we expect for our children and communicate quickly and honestly with families about how well their kids are meeting those targets.

For too long, such accountability has been considered in a negative light, but, in fact, it is an opportunity to better serve all students and to root out systemic issues that have put some at a

> *For too long, such accountability has been considered in a negative light, but in fact it is an opportunity to better serve all students and to root out systemic issues that have put some at a disadvantage.*

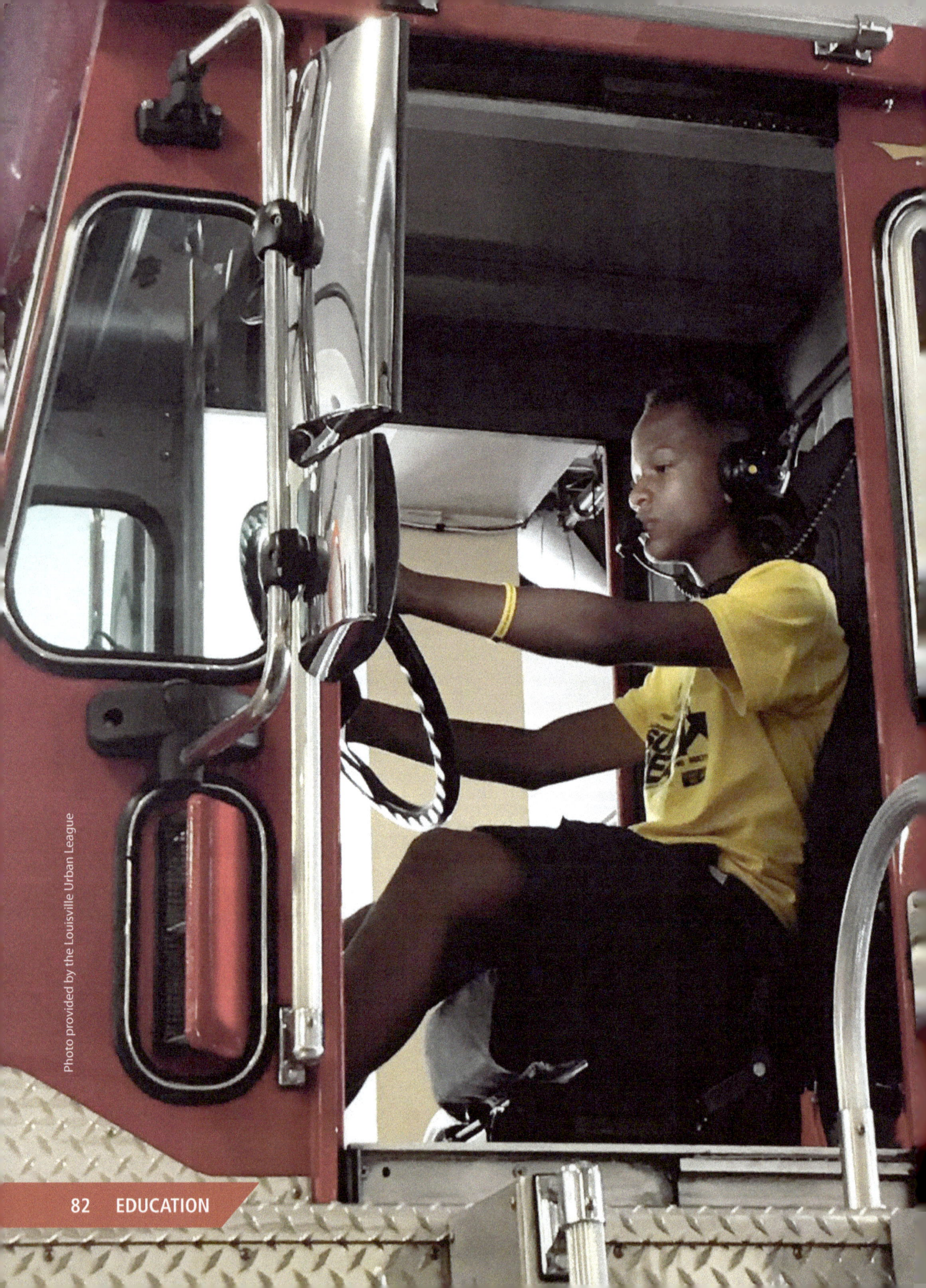

disadvantage. These efforts will be assisted by the fact that all indicators must be disaggregated by individual student subgroups including each major racial and ethnic group.

In that regard, design matters. If education standards are too complicated or incomprehensible, or if we lower the bar for the sake of giving the impression schools are doing better than they are, then we will waste this historic opportunity. That requires strong support for educators, pressure to encourage policymakers to do the right thing, and broad participation to tailor the system to our kids' needs. Most importantly, states must provide timely, transparent analysis of student performance for parents and communities in an easy-to-read, accessible format.

To be sure, that is a tall order. "This is going to be hard and intense work, but work that is needed," State Education Commissioner Stephen Pruitt wrote in July.[85] "We need all of our educators and shareholders to be engaged and willing to inform the process." We must push through bureaucracy and political gridlock to advocate on behalf of our children, because they can't wait.

Good enough is no longer good enough for our students.

Despite improvements in recent years, Kentucky continues to dwell in the basement of educational achievement. We need able-bodied, college- and career-ready high school graduates in order to attract quality companies and good paying jobs. It is with that understanding that we are working with Commissioner Pruitt to collect public input and create a system that takes care of children and ensures that every student succeeds.

Our work is also focused on creating stopgaps to ensure failing schools are identified and strategies are in place to help them turn around – effectively matching accountability with the right mix of muscle

and flexibility. Our system should be agile and adjustable when problems arise. But the expectation is clear: all schools must raise achievement for all students. That means:

► Ensuring schools are meeting expectations for all students and student subgroups, and that appropriate mechanisms are in place when schools do not meet those expectations;

► Highlighting and celebrating schools that meet and exceed expectations for groups they serve;

► Supporting leaders who are willing to direct necessary resources to struggling districts to help them improve;

► Requiring prompt, thorough, and competent responses for and from schools that need help; and

► Providing resources to help disadvantaged student groups achieve to high expectations.

Kentuckians have a historic opportunity to implement meaningful systems of accountability for all students. Achieving those goals will require strategic focus; we can't afford a watered-down plan that settles for "good enough."

THE EXPERIENCE OF YOUNG, GIFTED, AND BLACK STUDENTS IN JEFFERSON COUNTY PUBLIC SCHOOLS (JCPS)

Dr. Ahmad Washington, Assistant Professor
Department of Counseling and Human Development, University of Louisville

The Louisville Urban League remains steadfastly committed to the mission of providing Louisville's Black students with an equitable, intellectually rigorous, and holistically affirming education. Achieving educational equity for Black children in Louisville demands that we courageously name the anti-Black beliefs and practices that created and maintain educational inequality in Louisville and across the country.

In all honesty, this country has flourished socially, politically, and economically by legalizing the systematic miseducation and educational disenfranchisement of Black people.[86][87][88][89] In her groundbreaking text, "White Rage," Carol Anderson illustrates the ways in which the educational aspirations and economic prosperity of Black people have been historically intertwined, and why Whites have had a feverish investment in nullifying success in both domains.

Anderson discusses the roles that White local, state, and federal officials have repeatedly played in undermining Black people's efforts to achieve any semblance of agency and sociopolitical and economic self-sufficiency.[90] For instance, Anderson recounts stories in the early 1900s where White plantation owners flagrantly exploited Black sharecroppers by voiding agreements and refusing to pay them fair and livable wages for their physical labor. Emboldened by an indifferent legal system that scoffed at the notion of Black humanity, and with the support of vengeful White mobs who maimed and lynched Blacks for having the audacity to demand fair treatment, White plantation owners engaged in dishonest and unethical business practices towards Black sharecroppers with impunity.

It is in this context of racial domination that we also learn about the measures White plantation owners were willing to take to maximize profit at the expense of Black children's intellectual gifts. These measures included implementing an abbreviated school day and academic year to ensure that Black children would labor alongside their parents in the fields rather than learn valuable educational content. Fast forward to the 1950s and we find that little had changed for Black families. Whether it was housing covenants that prevented homeownership in the supposed liberal North and Midwest after the Great Migration or segregated and substandard academic environments for Black children under the blatant racial tyranny of the Jim Crow South, Black families encountered countless stumbling blocks as they sought employment opportunities and equitable educational facilities for Black children.

Contemporarily, we still see myriad instances where the educational welfare of Black children is treated with egregious disregard. Recently, it was revealed that several students and teachers in numerous Baltimore City Public Schools had to contend with freezing temperatures during the school day.[91] Angered by the unthinkable and deplorable conditions Baltimore children were expected to silently endure, several onlookers cynically asked how Baltimore, a city that opened a state-of-the-art, $35 million dollar youth detention center in September of 2017, could honestly proclaim in good faith that it does not have adequate funding to invest in education and other complimentary social service programs for the city's most marginalized youth.[92]

Similar frustrations have been articulated elsewhere across the country when Black children have been denied access to the educational resources they deserve. For instance, public outrage was swift and resounding when teachers documented how mold and mushrooms could be seen growing on the walls in one Detroit public school.[93] This type of chronic, systemic educational injustice and the impact it has had on the lives of Black children has been a topic of serious debate and discussion within education for quite some time.[94]

In other words, there has never been a time in this country's existence when cultivating the intellectual and artistic genius of Black children has been a priority. Instead, stereotypes about the purported intellectual inferiority of Black children or the cultural depravity of Black communities have been used to disallow Black children from accessing adequately funded, Whites only public schools, and to justify the gross psychological, emotional, and physical mistreatment of Black students.[95] [96]

Because educational inequities are the consequence of several converging factors, reversing educational inequity in Louisville for Black students will require herculean effort and strategic interventions. A complete and comprehensive list of interventions is beyond the scope of this piece; however, what follows is a brief list of suggestions that are informed by my own personal observations in various JCPS schools and personal anecdotes received from educators, parents, and Black students across the city. Based on these sources, educational equity for Black students in Louisville can germinate through:

▶ A more racially-diverse educator workforce that demonstrates unapologetic love for Black children;

▶ An anti-racist curriculum that affirms Black children; and

▶ A complete overhaul to disciplinary practices that disproportionately punish Black students.

THE NEED FOR A MORE DIVERSE EDUCATION WORKFORCE.
According to the U.S. Department of Education (2016), 82% of elementary and secondary public school teachers identify as White.[97] In JCPS, White women and White men comprise 46% and 40% of the high school teacher workforce, respectively.[98] Similarly, Bridgeland and Bruce (2011) found that 75% of the school counselors they surveyed nationally identified as White.[99] In JCPS, 60% of high school counselors are White women, while Black

women are sparsely represented at 16%. [100]

Increasing the pipeline to education for aspiring Black teachers – and other Black educators for that matter (e.g., school counselors, principals) – is important because having a Black teacher reduces the likelihood that a low-income Black student will drop out,[101] and decreases the frequency with which Black students experience suspensions and expulsions.[102] Funding to recruit, retain, and graduate future Black educators at institutions like the University of Louisville is something that must absolutely be prioritized if the mission is to provide an equitable education for Black students in Louisville.

MORE CULTURALLY-RELEVANT SCHOOL CURRICULUM.

The traditional American educational curriculum is designed to center and reproduce European thought and ideals and, at the same time, minimize and underappreciate the experiences, insights, and intellectual contributions of Black people.[103] [104] This curriculum is problematic because it fundamentally asks Black students to devalue and disavow their membership or proximity to their cultural group. [105] [106]

A revised curriculum – one that offers a more factual presentation of history – provides a more affirming depiction of Black life and helps Black children envision solutions to the problems we encounter as a

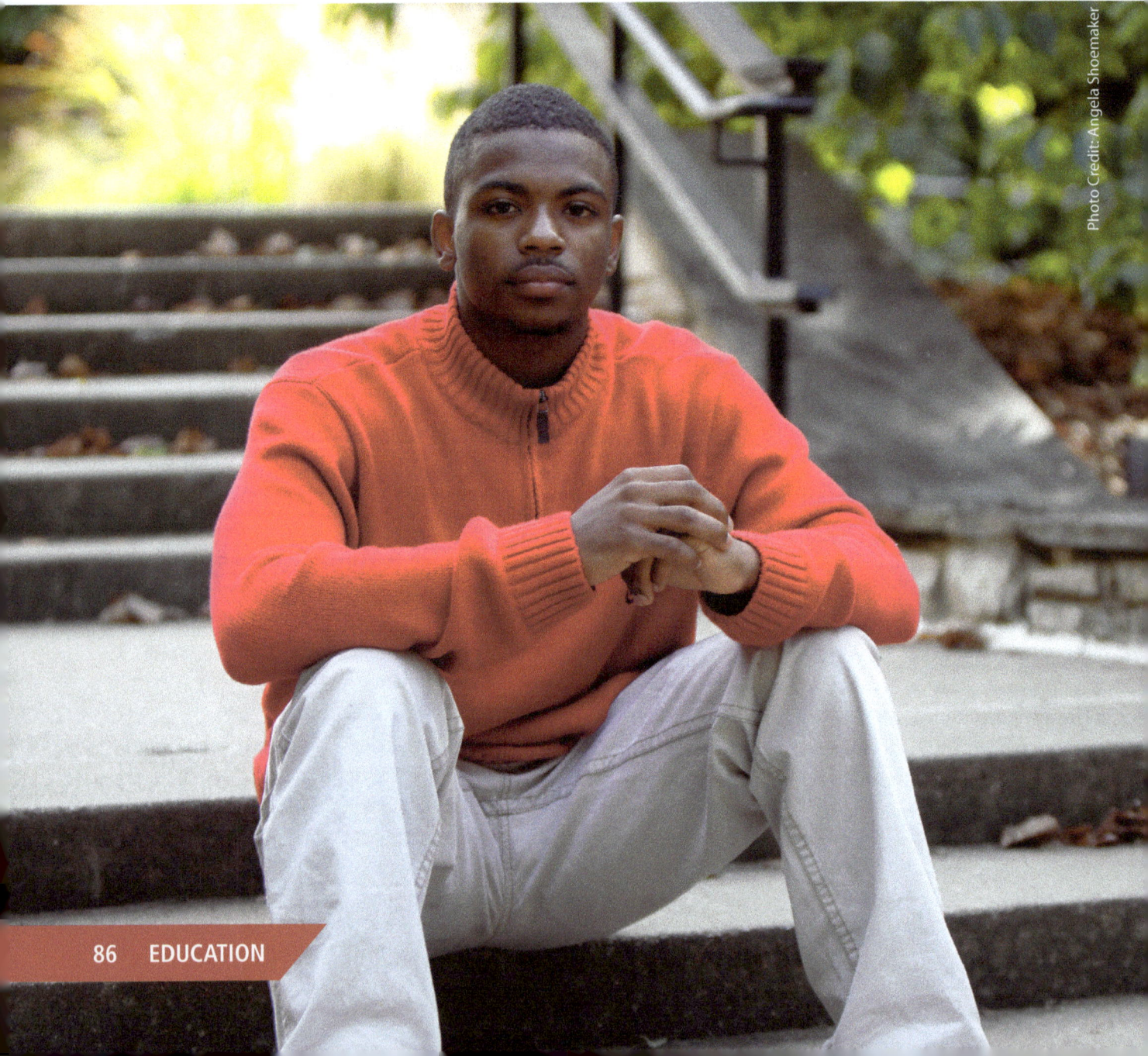

people. It is the type of culturally-relevant curriculum Black students across the country are clamoring to receive.[107] From this perspective, education should never just be about committing names, random dates and calculations to memory; instead, as Wade Nobles (1998) tells us, "education must be consciously guided by an awareness, understanding, and utilization of the historical conditions and cultural experiences which shape and give meaning to Black children's reality" (p. xv).[108] This radical vision of education has to be central in any legitimate discussion on equitable learning experiences for Black students in Louisville.

ENDING THE RELIANCE ON DISCIPLINE AND HYPERPOLICING IN SCHOOLS.

Perhaps no other issue represents a more pressing barrier to educational equity for the young, gifted, and Black students in JCPS than the frequency with which they are suspended and expelled. Data from the district reveal Black students are burdened by suspensions and expulsions at rates that far exceed their representation in the district.[109]

While some might subscribe to the racist belief that these data reflect Black children being hardwired or socialized culturally to be more disrespectful, oppositional, or physically violent towards school authority figures, evidence emphatically illustrates that Black students are penalized much harsher than their White classmates typically for violating subjective and vaguely-worded discipline policies (e.g., disrespect, noncompliance).[110] These disciplinary trends are born out of a deeply engrained ideology and system that characterizes Black children as deficient and inherently at-risk and, thus, treats them as disposable. We need newer, more humane educational frameworks that recognize, first and foremost, the insidious ways that institutional White supremacy constrains the lives of Black families and Black children and, second, how countless Black students navigate these obstacles to accomplish their aspirations.

If history is any indication, the mere articulation of recommendations like these will engender cynicism, apathy, and indignation from right and far-right White conservatives, as well as tepid support from White moderates and liberals. The incrementalism desired by the White moderate on matters like education reform is something Dr. King (1963) warned us about.[111] Shakur (1987) said, outright, that it would be asinine to expect the dominant educational system to "teach you your true history, teach you your true heroes, if they know that that knowledge will help set you free" (p. 181).[112]

Therefore, it is imperative that this community, the community we are all invested in, create alternative spaces where liberatory and transgressive learning occurs to supplement the schooling Black children are not receiving from the traditional K-12 pipeline.

MAKING POSTSECONDARY EDUCATION A REALITY: 55,000 DEGREES AND BEYOND

Mary Gwen Wheeler, Executive Director
Dr. Matt Berry, Director of Strategy & Impact
55,000 Degrees

The education attainment statistics are alarming and the trend lines are mostly in the wrong direction:

▶ In 2016, less than half (only 48%) of the Black students who graduated from Jefferson County Public Schools (JCPS) went on to attend a college or university in the next year.[113] That's down from 65% as recently as 2009.

▶ The gap in college-going between Black and White students is now nine points.[114] It was only three points in 2009.

▶ While high school graduation rates at JCPS are at a historic high for all demographic groups (80.6% overall),[115] that high school diploma does not mean the same thing for all students. In 2017, only 40% of African American graduates from JCPS were "college or career ready" compared to 71% for White graduates – a 30-point differential![116]

▶ When these gaps are stacked on each other, it is not surprising that only a quarter (24.4%) of working-age African American adults in Jefferson County have an associate's degree or higher, while almost half of Whites do (47.2%).[117]

This concern is not merely "academic." When education beyond high school is more important than ever, the downward trend in college-going rates is not good for our economy nor for our young people's futures.

By 2020, at least 60% of the jobs in Kentucky will require a postsecondary degree, according to estimates from the Georgetown University's Center on Education and the Workforce (CEW).[118] Moreover, 75% of the family-supporting jobs projected to be added in Louisville by the middle of the 2020s will require at least some postsecondary education, including community and technical college –

according to a joint report by KentuckianaWorks and 55,000 Degrees.[119]

The challenge before us is to make college education an opportunity, not a perpetuator of the historic divides. Assessment and college access should open up opportunity rather than certifying existing inequities or validating privileges of class and race as meritocracy.

To change these racialized outcomes, we must get to the root causes including poverty and its effects on school performance, the lingering effects of systemic racism, and the question of college affordability.

Let's look at these three issues:

POVERTY AND READINESS

As the essay provided by 15,000 Degrees outlines, the "readiness" gap at the end of high school starts much earlier, even in kindergarten. Poverty tied to race is obvious, with 45% of Black children in Louisville living in poverty, compared to 14% of White children.[120] When needs of poor kids are not addressed, they do not thrive in the classroom. In the end, too many African American students are led to believe that postsecondary education is not for them and too many begin to internalize this, starting as early as middle school, thinking that they "are not college material."

LINGERING SYSTEMIC RACISM

In Kentucky, we are only a couple generations removed from the effects of the Day Law of 1904, which excluded Blacks from accessing public or private White colleges or universities. Dr. Kevin Cosby, President of Simmons College, recently told us that his father was restricted to the segregated division of the University of Louisville until 1951. That explicit racism may seem to be a part of the past, but it still affects students today. First-generation Black students, particularly low-income students, face particular challenges in paying for college and staying on track once enrolled. In 2015, the six-year graduation rate at our local four-year institutions was 34% for Black students and the three-year graduation rate at local two-year institutions was in the single digits at 8%![121]

COLLEGE AFFORDABILITY

The average in-state tuition at Kentucky's public colleges and universities has grown from about $5,000 per year to about $8,900 per year. That's an 81% increase. In that same time period, the price at public two-year institutions in the state went up almost 60%.[122]

All three of these factors reinforce and play into each other. That's why 55,000 Degrees is taking part in a transformative new partnership called Louisville Promise. At the center of the promise will be a scholarship fund, the goal of which is to ensure that every JCPS graduate can afford at least two years of community or technical college. We know, however, that the challenge goes much deeper than money and so our partnership of public and private agencies will work together and work smarter to deliver the opportunities and supports that every student needs to be successful.

Louisville Promise is not a traditional solution to the policies and practices that have plagued us for generations. It is a new way of doing business that acknowledges our past and lends the support of an entire community toward building a better future. Join us, and go to *www.louisvillepromise.org* to share your dreams.

RESHAPING THE JCPS EDUCATIONAL CURRICULUM TO FIT A MORE ACCURATE REPRESENTATION OF THE STUDENT DEMOGRAPHICS

John Marshall, Chief Equity Officer
Jefferson County Public Schools

When we look at the state of Black Louisville as it relates to education, it is clear that the systemic inequities that contribute to the debilitation of Black Louisville outside of the schoolhouse play a role in the inequities inside the schoolhouse. Further, when one looks at the performance data tied to Black students, it does not take deep scientific scrutiny to see that there are gaps betwixt Black students and their peers. For the sake of parsimony, the two gaps to which I will unpack are the following: lack of participation in gifted and talented programming, and hegemonic curriculum.

To be clear, systemic racism is the kindle that ignites this bond fire of belittlement and performance outcomes. There is no other way to explain the unexplainable and unacceptable outcomes befallen too many of our students.

For the 2017-2018 school year, Jefferson County Public Schools (JCPS) has 34,797 Black students enrolled in kindergarten through 12th grade.[123] Over the last 24 months, the public school system in Louisville has become a majority-minority school district, meaning that the majority of the students that the public school system serves are non-White. There is an opportunity in that shift.

Along with the recent demographic changes, JCPS could "colorize" the curriculum to reflect the majority non-White clientele it serves. It is clear and research-proven that curricula impacts the sense of belonging and furthers the psychology of students of color. The messaging behind the curriculum does not speak to the greatness of African [Americans]. In fact, it attempts and is often successful, although highly inaccurate, at convincing the Black learner that our lateness to the world stage is in fact accurate.

In the 2017-18 school year, the majority of students in

JCPS were performing at a "Novice" and "Apprentice" level in reading and math.[124] In addition, according to the Jefferson County's latest Envision Equity scorecard, Black students did not feel as if they belonged to the school. To be clear, this sentiment was not just held/endured by Blacks that are living in poverty. The same sentiment was shared by middle-class and affluent Blacks.

The state of Black Louisville as it relates to education sits juxtaposed to exclusive curricula that struggles to invite the new majority of the learners into the lesson in a manner that equitably and accurately applauds the contributions, commitment, and brightness of its darker-hued learners. To that end, it is also clear that curricula corrupts absolutely. The prescriptive pedagogy and curriculum that inoculates the very malleable mind of Black students shackles the psyche and lynches metacognitive aptitudes. Further, one must investigate and argue that curriculum and pedagogy influences (mis)behaviors and fortifies the marginalization of many.

Recognizing that the majority of students are now non-White, JCPS is still disproportionate in the percentage of Black students identified and participating in the Gifted and Talented program. Fifty-six percent of JCPS students are of color while Black students only represent 8.7% (2,873 students) participating in Gifted and Talented.[125] As JCPS addresses this facet of disproportionality, the school system and the community must take heed to the unspoken and (maybe) unintended statement that is being made by this fact. Further, as we focus on culture and climate, there must be a powerful look at what that means.

The systemic and historical vestiges of redlining, slavery, curricular gentrification, systemic (endemic) racism, and White supremacy impact all aspects of the (school) system. Just like infractions such as disruptive behavior (which has been removed from the JCPS Student Support and Behavior Intervention[126]) and failure to obey are subjective, so is, in many cases, the consideration of giftedness. Consequently, giftedness and access to the

Photo provided by the Louisville Urban League

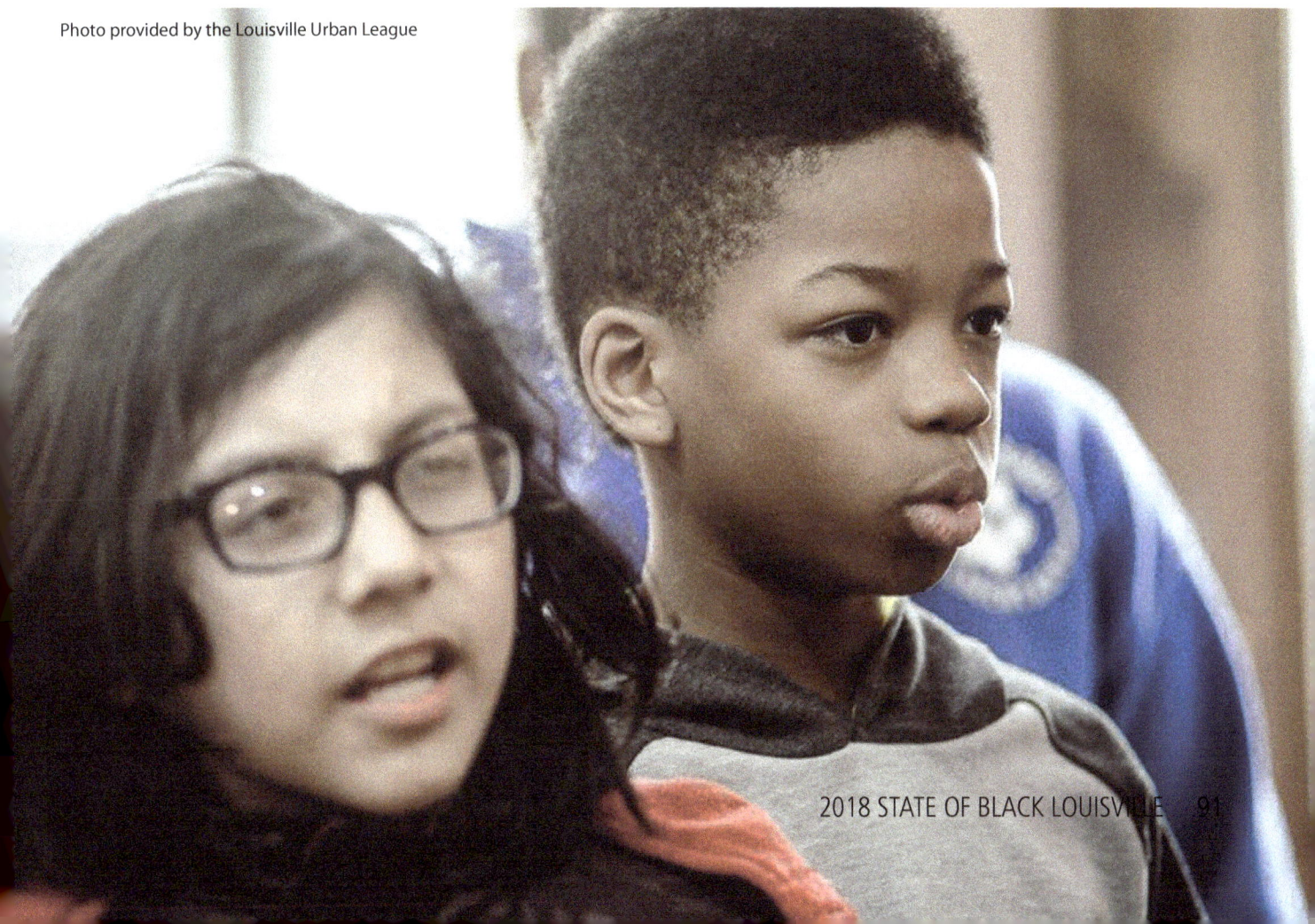

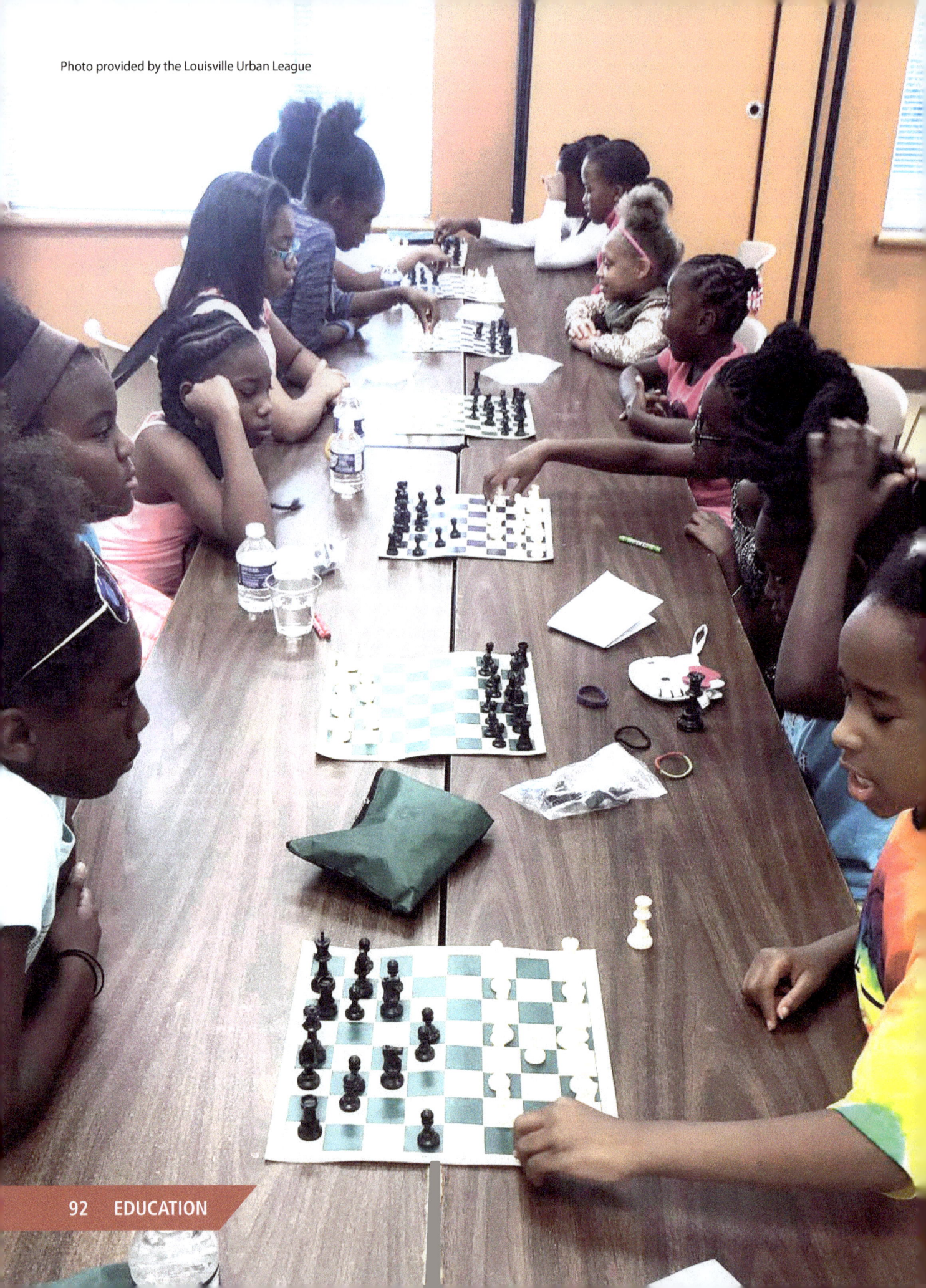

advanced-level course work is limited to few Blacks.

Louisville, Kentucky must question the profound and longstanding practices that gentrify curriculum. We must also demand that the cognitive and cultural gifts that Black children possess get recognized and protected. To that point, the subjectivity and low expectations mind-cuffs the mind of many Black students.

The following is a recommendation Louisville needs to do in order to address this very fluid and intentional system:

Create policy that obliterates the systemic inequities that are facing Black students. Said policy should:

- ▶ Create an auxiliary community group that accurately scrutinizes the actions of JCPS as it relates to diversity, equity, and addressing poverty.

- ▶ Mandate that staffs reflect the demographic of the city (providing time to reach that goal).

- ▶ Partner with Pan-African Studies of the University of Louisville to do an overhaul in masse of the historical content taught to students.

- ▶ Partner with teachers that demonstrate an understanding and proficient utility of imbedding inclusive anti-racist curriculum.

- ▶ Redesign the entire K-12 curriculum to include the greatness of African [Americans]. This curriculum should be sociopolitical, culturally relevant, and historically inclusive.

- ▶ Require all teachers and staff to receive mandatory cultural competence training from experts locally and nationally on a yearly basis.

- ▶ Require that all schools have the same rigorous levels of course offerings.

- ▶ Require that Black students are equally reflected in the gifted and talented programs.

- ▶ Staff/place principals in buildings according to disposition and cultural and climatic understanding of the school and community to which he/she serves.

Insist that teacher preparation programs train aspiring teachers to understand, utilize, and address sociopolitical constructs, cultural differences, racism, and educational equity explicitly in their classroom.

- ▶ Audit the syllabi of all colleges of education in Louisville.

- ▶ Create courses that focus on educational equity:

- ▶ Cultural competence in the urban classroom

- ▶ Racism and the effects on teaching and learning

- ▶ Culturally-competent curriculum design

- ▶ Critical Race Theory (Hip Hop, politics, anti-racism, anti-sexism)

The state of Black Louisville cannot solely be attributed to Black Louisvillians. State, by definition, is the condition that someone or something is in at a particular time. These conditions were not shaped by Black America (Louisville); thus, these conditions should not be blamed on Black America (Louisville). We must look at practices and policies, or the lack thereof, that proliferate and safeguard a system that was not designed for or by us.

YOUTH INVESTMENT MUST BE A PRIORITY

Timothy E. Findley, Jr., Pastor
Kingdom Fellowship Christian Life Center

I believe without a shadow of doubt that we will all benefit most when every child has the opportunity to grow up to become truly remarkable, to contribute his or her special gifts and talents to the future economic and social vitality of our community. Every parent sees endless possibilities and great hope in the eyes of a child. As a city, when we look at our children, we see tomorrow's leaders — scientists, teachers, doctors, and change agents. For our children to thrive, though, we must support their development

The future starts here, with all our children who deserve nothing less. We must invest in their most essential tools. What are the most essential tools? Their brains, their hearts, and their physical health. Our collective commitment to the next generation must begin before the first day of school. Our commitment to our children must become a priority.

The future vitality of our city will require investments in human capital.

Studies offer concrete statistics that proper investments improve classroom behavior, school attendance, academic aspirations, and reduce the tendency toward dropping out and drug use. There are even studies showing a reduction in criminal behavior, lower instances of obesity, and greater physical activity. The success of communities, businesses, and the economy depend on preparing our children for the challenges of the next century. Deploying the wisest funding strategies to convert "day care center" to robust and available "early learning centers," and to fully fund after-school programs for all our children, helps to get us there. But, to succeed in the overall mission, we must collectively invest in our children and secure the dedicated commitment of communities, businesses and, most of all, our elected officials at every level.

Like all states, Kentucky faces tough financial decisions as it works to balance its budget and wisely spend taxpayer money. However, investing in early childhood education is a no-brainer. Not only is it a question of equal opportunity for kids, but research from Nobel Prize-winning economist James Heckman shows that investments in high-quality programs can yield an annual 13 percent return, per child, per year, through improved outcomes such as reduced crime,

higher graduation rates, and improved sociability.[127]

The future vitality of our city will require investments in human capital. The current challenge is to target strategic investments in our children during the years when their potential is greatest. This must become a community priority.

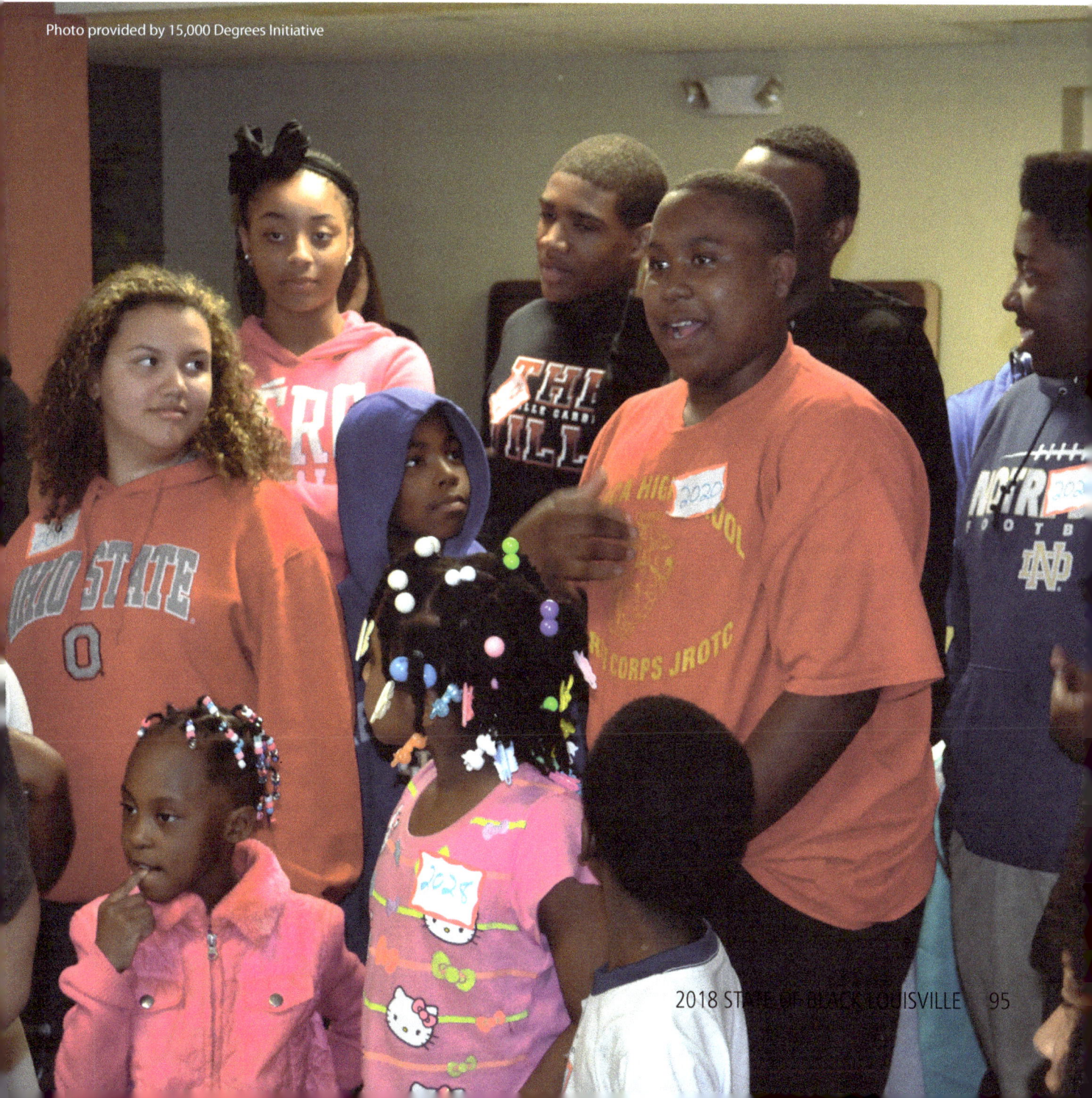

Photo provided by 15,000 Degrees Initiative

CHALLENGES TO BLACK ACCESS TO HIGHER EDUCATION IN KENTUCKY

Dr. Ricky L. Jones, Professor and Chair
Department of Pan-African Studies, University of Louisville

Late in 2017, Gov. Matt Bevin and the General Assembly approved yet another in a long line of cuts to higher education funding in Kentucky. This one a scathing 4.5 percent. The state's political leaders argued this was necessary in order to deal with underfunded state workers' pensions. While the pension crisis is real, Kentucky's continuing lack of commitment to higher education can lead to no good.

Disturbingly, Democrats *and* Republicans have been equally committed to financially gutting the state's institutions of higher learning for years. Linda Blackford of the Lexington Herald-Leader cites a Washington-based "Center on Budget and Policy Priorities" (CBPP) report in concluding, "Kentucky has made some of the deepest cuts to higher education in the country since 2008 (over 26 percent), putting it among the 10 states with the biggest per-student funding reductions for public universities and community colleges." It is also one of only 13 states that has continued to cut state funding to higher education between 2016 and 2017.

This is a disquieting trend in a state that is already one of the most undereducated in America. U.S. Census data ranks Kentucky 45th in percentage of citizens 25 or older with high school diplomas. It ranks a dismal 47th in percentage of people with bachelor's degrees. Only Mississippi, Arkansas, and West Virginia are worse.

The question is, will Kentucky's leaders listen or stay on a course that continues to create an increasingly dumbed down citizenry?

The CBPP points out that higher education disinvestment has profoundly negative consequences, "The funding decline has contributed to higher tuition and reduced quality on campuses as colleges have had to balance budgets by reducing faculty, limiting course offerings, and in some cases closing campuses. At a time when the benefit of a college education has never been greater, state policymakers have made going to college less affordable and less accessible to the students most in need."

Kenny Colston, spokesman for the "Kentucky Center for Economic Policy", laments, "This report shows that as the majority of states are re-investing in their futures by committing to funding higher education (in the decade after the Great Recession), Kentucky continues to move in the wrong direction. Every cut in state funding puts pressure on students by resulting in rising tuition costs — which prices low-income students out of opportunities and forces thousands of others into unmanageable student loan debt."

Considering that blacks are disproportionately poor, undereducated, underrepresented in higher education upper administrative positions, faculties, and student populations – these facts are particularly troubling.

CBPP advises, "State lawmakers must renew their commitment to high-quality, affordable public higher education by increasing the revenue these schools receive. By doing so, they can help build a stronger middle class and develop the entrepreneurs and skilled workers needed for a strong state economy." The question is, will Kentucky's leaders listen or stay on a course that continues to create an increasingly dumbed down citizenry? To do so would only maintain structures that benefit a small number of ruling elites by reifying long-standing social, educational, political, economic, and racial stratification. Louisville, the state's greatest economic and intellectual engine, would remain a city where members of the same four or five wealthy groups enjoy never-ending power, influence, and access

while the rest degenerate.

It's clear this continued defunding of higher education isn't just about the pension crisis. Contradictions abound. Louisville Mayor Greg Fischer opined, "It doesn't make sense to consider cuts that can hurt a child's classroom, law enforcement, drug treatment or our justice system when we don't tax country club members and limousine rides – that's just not right."

To be sure, this is serious. Thriving cities and states have thriving universities. Poor ones do not. At the end of the day, Kentucky has to decide what it wants to be in the most multiracial, multiethnic, multicultural, and increasingly educated America we have seen to date. Are thoroughbreds, bourbon, and basketball more important than brains? Does it wish to be a state that develops cosmopolitan, 21st century sensibilities where smart people want to visit and live or will it continue to be a backwards-thinking, clannish anachronism? Will it grow its educated class and invest in the future or continue glorifying anti-intellectualism, celebrating mediocrity, and rallying around confederate statutes and all their accoutrements? Only time will tell. No matter what happens, blacks in Louisville will be greatly impacted.

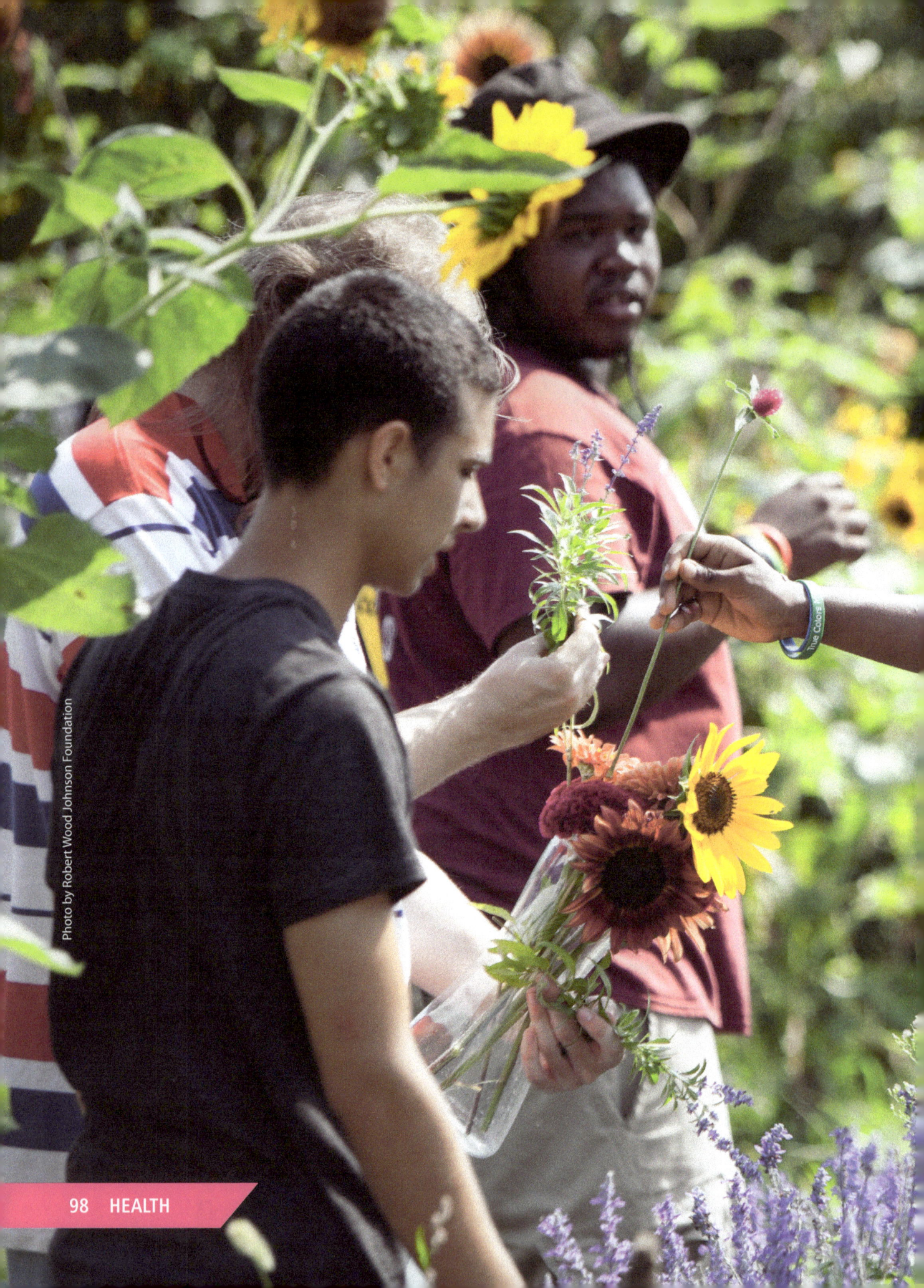

Photo by Robert Wood Johnson Foundation

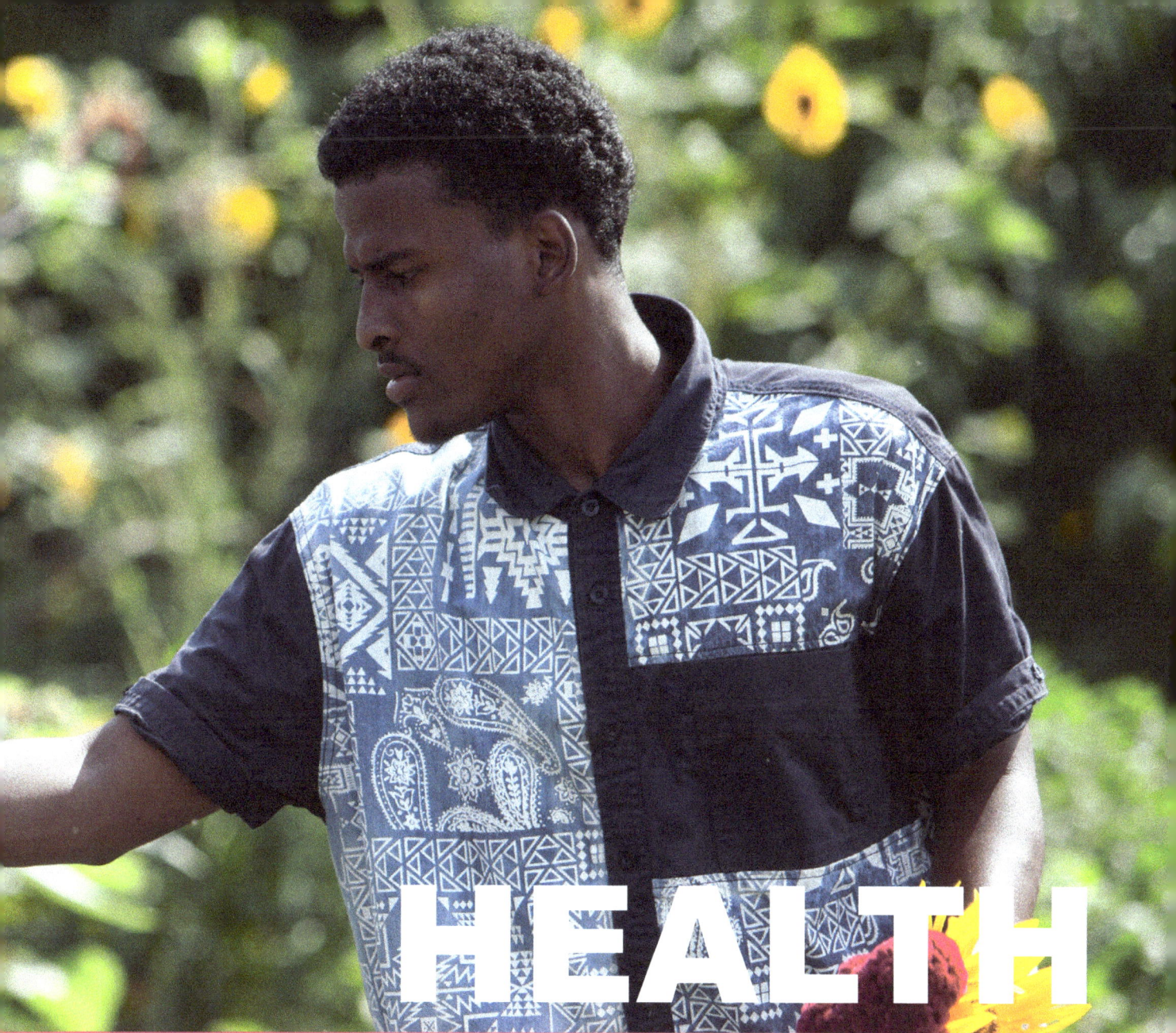

HEALTH

The city should collaborate with the local Urban League and appropriate health care facilities to enhance community education on health and wellness issues. The racial disparities in health care need to be broadly exposed in our community. We should encourage and expand a healthy city campaign to ensure that affordable, high-quality health care is available to all residents. Healthy lifestyles and high-quality health care should be viewed as a human right, not as a privilege available only to those who can afford access to quality health care.

Lastly, we cannot ignore the devastating drug epidemic in our community. We must seek additional resources from state and federal government for drug prevention and treatment programs.

John J. Johnson, Executive Director
Kentucky Commission on Human Rights

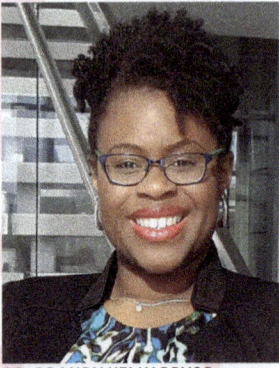

DR. BRANDY KELLY PRYOR, University of Louisville

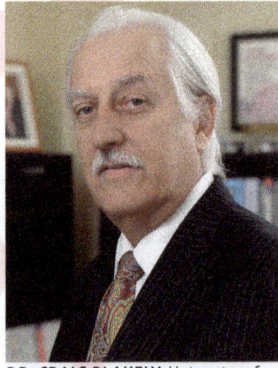

DR. CRAIG BLAKELY, University of Louisville

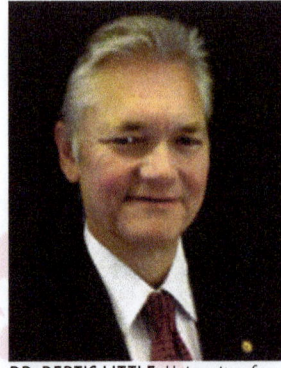

DR. BERTIS LITTLE, University of Louisville

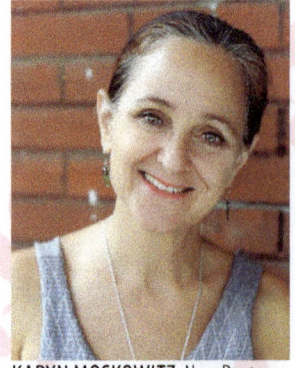

KARYN MOSKOWITZ, New Roots, Inc.

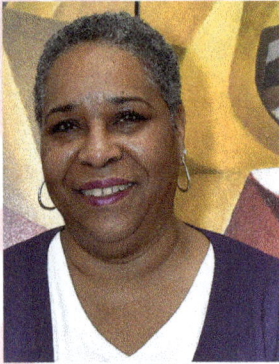

MARY MONTGOMERY, New Roots, Inc.

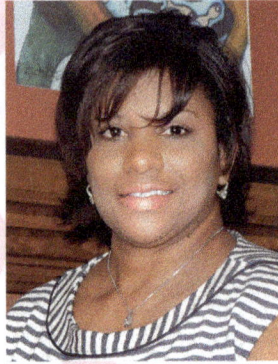

YVETTE GENTRY, Metro United Way

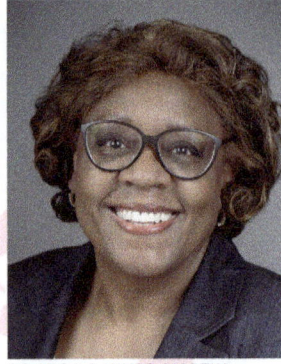

DR. VICKI P. HINES-MARTIN, University of Louisville

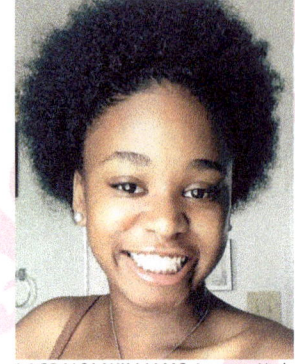

LAGRAICA WILLIAMS, Iroquois High School

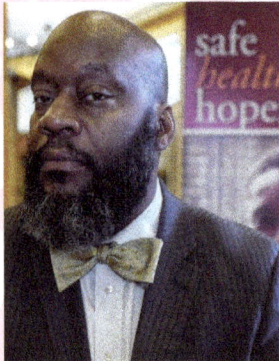

ANTHONY SMITH, Cities United

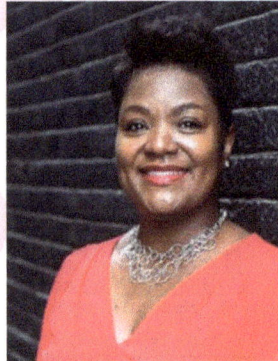

SADIQA N. REYNOLDS, ESQ., Louisville Urban League

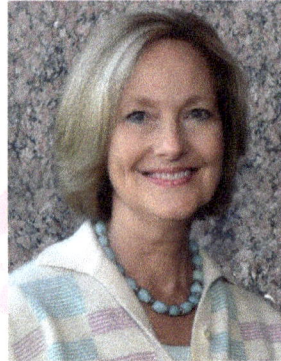

VIRGINIA KELLY JUDD, The Humana Foundation

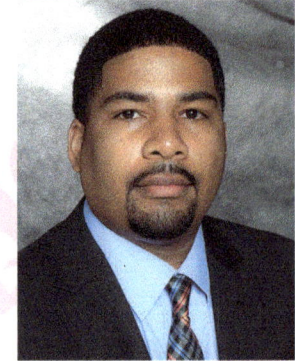

DR. ARMON R. PERRY, University of Louisville

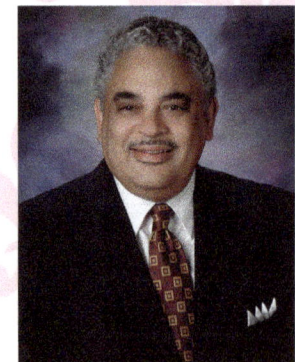

JOHN J. JOHNSON, Kentucky Commission on Human Rights

NOTHING CAN BE CHANGED, UNTIL IT IS FACED: A LOOK AT HEALTH EQUITY IN BLACK LOUISVILLE

Brandy N. Kelly Pryor, PhD, Assistant Professor; Director
University of Louisville
Center for Health Equity, Louisville Metro Public Health and Wellness

Battling racism and battling heterosexism and battling apartheid share the same urgency inside me as battling cancer. None of these struggles are ever easy, and even the smallest victory is never taken for granted. . ."
- Audre Lorde, 1986

For over a decade, the Center for Health Equity (CHE) at the Louisville Metro Department of Public Health and Wellness (LMPHW) has challenged the prevailing idea that health and disease are merely a result of individual behaviors. For centuries, inequitable laws, policies, and practices, derived from White supremacist thought, have shaped systems of power. These systems of power have shaped community well-being, resulting in overwhelming differences in *how well* and *how long* one may live. Dismantling these inequitable systems has been the unflinching goal of the Center for the past eleven years.

Recognizing James Baldwin's infamous claim, "… nothing can be changed until it is faced," CHE's Health Equity Report (HER) uses data to show how place and social systems matter to life outcomes. In breaking down the data by race, gender, location, and age, we can understand how the trauma of structural and institutional discrimination impacts life outcomes. The HER is a critical tool to provide evidence that health is a community problem and we must work together to change these outcomes and create a thriving future for all.

From cradle to grave, the 2017 Health Equity Report[128] shows that the intersection between race, gender, and age are having an impact on the health of Black Louisvillians:

► Infant health can have a lasting impact on

one's overall health later in life so it is critical to know that preterm births and low birth weight disproportionately affect Black babies. In addition, while infant mortality has slowly been falling in Louisville, the death rate for Black babies from 2011-2015 is nearly 2.5 times higher than for White babies and nearly 3 times higher than for Hispanic/Latino babies.

This inequity in infant health outcomes is a national phenomenon that has been strongly linked to the stress and consequences of racism. Studies show that even when education, marital, and income status are otherwise equal for Black mothers and White mothers, Black babies are disproportionately affected. Nevertheless, we do know that implementing paid parental leave policies for working parents and establishing funding to subsidize healthy foods is helpful for pregnant mothers, a healthy delivery, and the health of the infant.

▶ Violence, particularly homicide, is geographically concentrated in the northwestern areas of Jefferson County, meaning that certain communities are disproportionately experiencing the chronic stress of community violence. The group that is most affected is Black men, whose death rates from homicide are 5.5 times that of the Louisville Metro rate.

For many communities that have to navigate the structural and institutional consequences of economic divestment in their neighborhoods, poverty then isolates these communities socially and geographically from economically thriving communities. As a result, we often see violence as a mechanism for navigating economics and safety. Implementing programs to aid in wealth building and investing in the built environment and quality business and economic development in the neighborhood can have an impact on this health outcome.

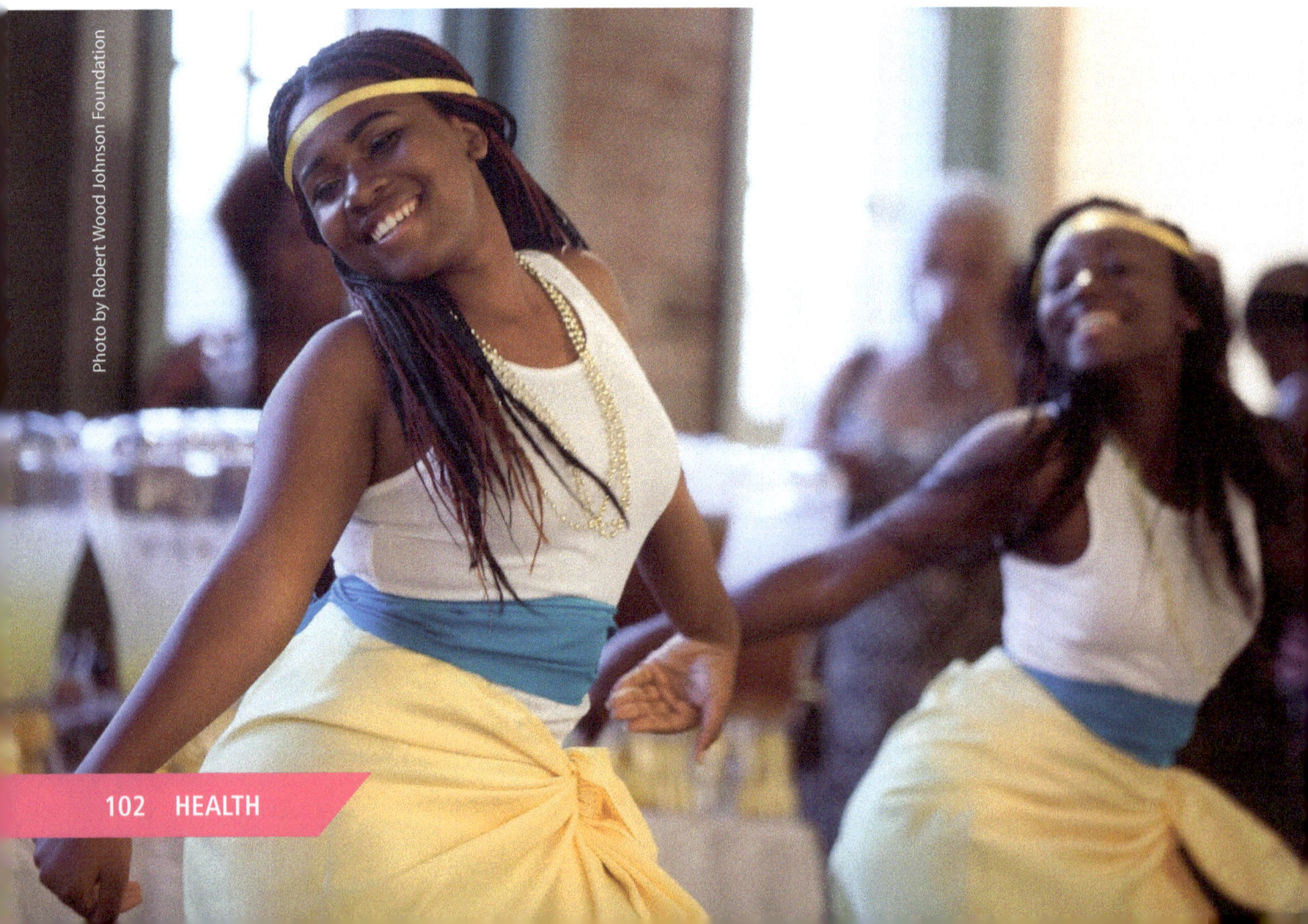

Photo by Robert Wood Johnson Foundation

- In Louisville, Black girls have some of the most alarming rates of diagnosis with chlamydia, gonorrhea, or syphilis – sexually transmitted infections (STIs) that can have long-term health outcomes. In 2015, Black girls were diagnosed with an STI at rates that were 2.76 times higher than Black boys, 5.06 times higher than White girls, and 26.7 times higher than White boys. It is important when looking at these vast differences in rates to not draw harmful and false conclusions about the individual sexual behaviors of Black girls but, rather, to demand more critical attention and research focusing on the structural and institutional barriers causing such harm. Although it is hard to draw causation for why rates are so high among Black girls, we do know there is a relationship between limited income and higher rates of sexually transmitted diseases (STDs) while those who live in neighborhoods with strong social supports, low mental distress, and less violence are at much lower risk.

Many solutions exist to aid in wealth building and alleviate the stress poverty such as implementing a state-level Earned Income Tax Credit. Additionally, we know that when young people are exposed to school-based health programs and have more access to health and human service providers in their neighborhoods, they are less likely to engage in activity that may cause them to be diagnosed with an STD.

- Death rates due to stroke and diabetes are 1.42 and 1.73 times higher, respectively, for Black Louisvillians compared to White counterparts. Black men are 1.2 times more likely to die of heart disease than White men, and Black women are 1.25 times more likely to die of it than White women. Additionally, Black men are 1.17 times more likely to die of cancer than White men, and Black women are 1.14 times more likely to die of cancer

than White women. Each of these health outcomes is exacerbated by a lack of access to healthy foods and health and human service providers.

- Given these disparities in death rates, Black men are expected to live 3.5 to 16.75 less years than men of other races. Black women are expected to live 2 to 12.72 less years than women of other races.

While the data presented here, and in the full 2017 Health Equity Report, is alarming, it does not provide a complete picture; the fragmented information we have are merely pieces of a much larger puzzle. For example, we are not able to show how our community members experience health outcomes by sexual orientation or beyond the gender binary of female and male. We also know that many of these health outcomes listed above are interconnected and the earlier in life one may experience one of these health outcomes it makes maintaining overall health throughout life more difficult. Overall, we must change the way we collect, analyze, and report data if we ever hope to find equitable solutions to these grave inequities and their root causes.

For each of the highlighted points above there are many root causes, such as neighborhood development, quality and affordability of housing, the criminal justice system, transportation and food accessibility, and our environmental quality, to name just a few. One of the most critical root causes is employment and income and how individuals are able to build wealth and assets over time to aid in the future development of their health and the generations that follow.

Discussion about these root causes and subsequent solutions can be found in the full Health Equity Report at www.healthequityreport.com. These solutions are listed for each health outcome as "best practices" and are assembled from comprehensive research that has assessed and evaluated policies and programs from around the country.

We know for solutions to work we need interventions at multiple levels of society, from the individual to community to the policy level, to make sustainable and long-term change for health. Whether we are trying to reduce infant mortality, homicides, transmission of STDs or death rates from chronic diseases, we need to ensure more opportunities for wealth-building, education and employment in our community for those that need it the most.

We cannot have a flourishing Louisville without a thriving Black Louisville: a Louisville where Black women and girls are fully cared for and accepted in their own right, not simply in relation to their male or White counterparts; where the health of Black men and boys is promoted through a lens of wellness instead of a state of crisis; and a city where our LGBTQ population, across race and class, is recognized as full and equal participants in our society.

A flourishing Louisville is one that challenges systems of power and oppression with all community voices at the table, no matter their identities. A flourishing Louisville speaks truthfully to the economically and politically powerful, and where leaders do not simply call for more acts of service from the public while failing to challenge the very systems they control and benefit from. A healthy Louisville is a just and equitable Louisville – not just for some, but for all.

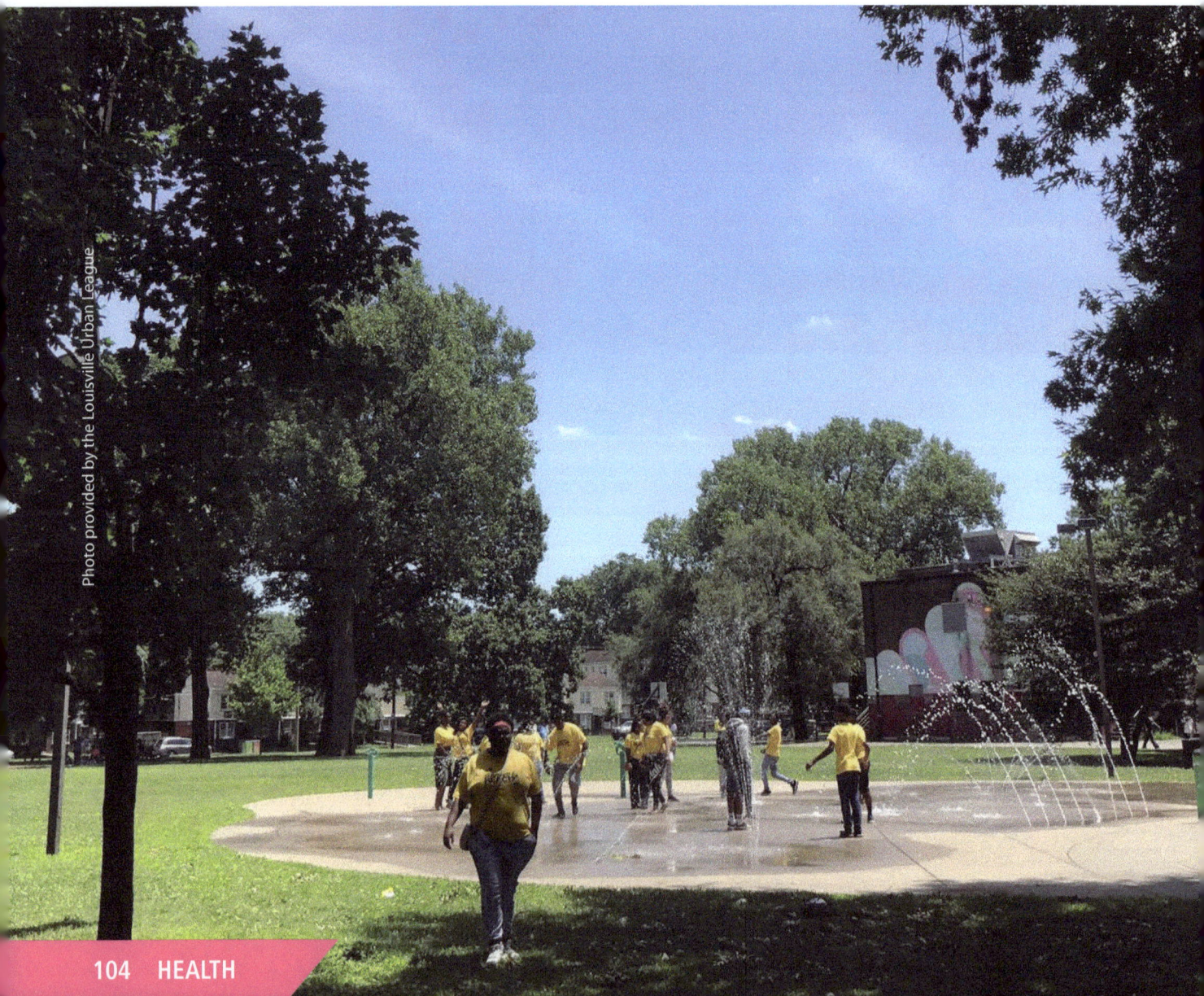

Photo provided by the Louisville Urban League

THE STATE OF BLACK LOUISVILLE: THE HEALTH PERSPECTIVE

Dr. Craig Blakely, Dean
Dr. Bertis Little, Professor

School of Public Health and Information Sciences, University of Louisville

It is alarming to observe that one can travel two miles west of City Hall or three miles east and find such extremely disparate characteristics that describe residents' homes, jobs, toys, hopes, aspirations and, simply, health. Residents of west Louisville (largely considered west of 9th Street and north of Algonquin Parkway), approximately 85,000,[129] face substantial health, social, educational, and economic difficulties compared to the remainder of Louisville metropolitan area. West Louisville is extremely segregated: more than 78% of its residents are African American[130] and more than 60% live in poverty. By comparison, less than 5% of White residents of east Louisville live in poverty.[131]

The best single indicator of a population's health and well-being is life expectancy. This simple indicator incorporates influences from birth through old age, including health, social, educational, and economic factors – all influenced by individual behavior, but more heavily linked to the sociopolitical factors that impact us in a myriad of ways.

In the mainly African American West End, life expectancy (genders combined) is approximately 67 years. By comparison, gender-combined life expectancy is 82 years in the eastern half of Jefferson County, which is more than 70% White. [132]

The facts are indisputable: being Black in west Louisville is detrimental to your health.

What is truly disheartening is that these differential death rates are fundamentally preventable. As can be seen in the table below,[133] [134] largely preventable causes of death contribute directly to this disparity.

These figures highlight the fact that both preventable diseases as well as culturally-influenced behaviors

TABLE 1. CAUSES OF DEATH*

	West Louisville	East Louisville
Alcohol and drug-related causes	21.4	3.0
Diabetes	82.0	13.0
Heart disease	341.0	120
Cancer	347.0	142
HIV/AIDS	30.0	0.5
Stroke	82.0	27.0
Homicide	68.0	0.5
Suicide	20.0	5.0
Accidents	73.0	20.0
Infant mortality	14.2	7.1

per 100,000 population

TABLE 2. SOCIAL DETERMINANTS BY ECONOMIC INDICATORS

	West Louisville	East Louisville
No Health Insurance	>25%	<10%
Percent of children in poverty	>95%	<5%
High school graduation percent	<25%	>95%
Unemployment	>25%	<5%
Lack reliable transportation	>50%	<5%
Percent of income spent on housing	>45%	<25%
Dilapidated housing (pre-1950's)	>70%	<5%
Vacant and abandoned housing	>7%	<1%
Violent crimes/year	>2500	<75

vary widely by community. The social determinants of health affect these mortality rates and their disparities. Jobs, education, housing, transportation, and income are determinants. The foundation of a history of policies and practices that provide differential access to our society's resources for disadvantaged segments of our population are also the principal determinants of these disparities.

One can further examine these social determinants by exploring differential access to common goods, those resources that we believe to be the right of all citizens – at least on paper. The second table[135][136] provides formal evidence of the differential access to these common goods across different segments of our community.

West Louisville was once home to a thriving African American community. Today, while we can find many examples of successful African American families, the residents of west Louisville do not comprise a thriving community on most metrics we know and value. Far too many suffer from constrained access to the lifestyles to which we all aspire and this directly and indirectly influences health status.

We had a great vision of a better country in the 1950s and '60s. It was an era characterized by protest. It was a time of life-altering policy initiatives that targeted access to education, anti-poverty programs, equal access to housing, and direct health care access. Yet here we are a half-century later, with limited evidence of meaningful changes in disparities in health indicators. Louisville, despite the efforts of many to transform our community, remains but another picture of failure on this front.

We need to continue to strive to provide a level playing field for all of our residents, for the entire community and all its members will only benefit from a more educated, more engaged work force and healthier population. These health disparities have existed in this country since its founding. Reducing racial/ethnic health disparities have been national health goals for decades and very little progress has been made. The fix is not just a function of differential access to care. The problem is much more complex and is rooted in the social determinants of health.

Frankly, the problem is us. As former U.S. President Barack Obama tweeted in response to the White supremacy march in Charlottesville, Virginia in

2017, quoting Nelson Mandela, "No one is born hating another person because of the color of his skin…"[137] Paraphrasing, none of us are born with the biases that create and maintain differential access to all the resources that contribute to these health disparities. We are taught the subtle and not-so-subtle ways to maintain the titled playing field that is "living while Black". The problem is, too many of those "driving the bus" – our teachers, our clergy, our police, our elected officials, the judiciary, and our parents – are carriers of the biases that perpetuate the issue.

The fix lies with the reactions of policymakers and the public to the Colin Kaepernicks of the world, those counter-protesting a racially-motivated free speech rally in Boston, and in the ballot boxes of Louisville. If we as individuals fail to recognize the source of the problem and do not proactively participate in the solution, then we are complicit with the problem.

Photo provided by the Louisville Urban League

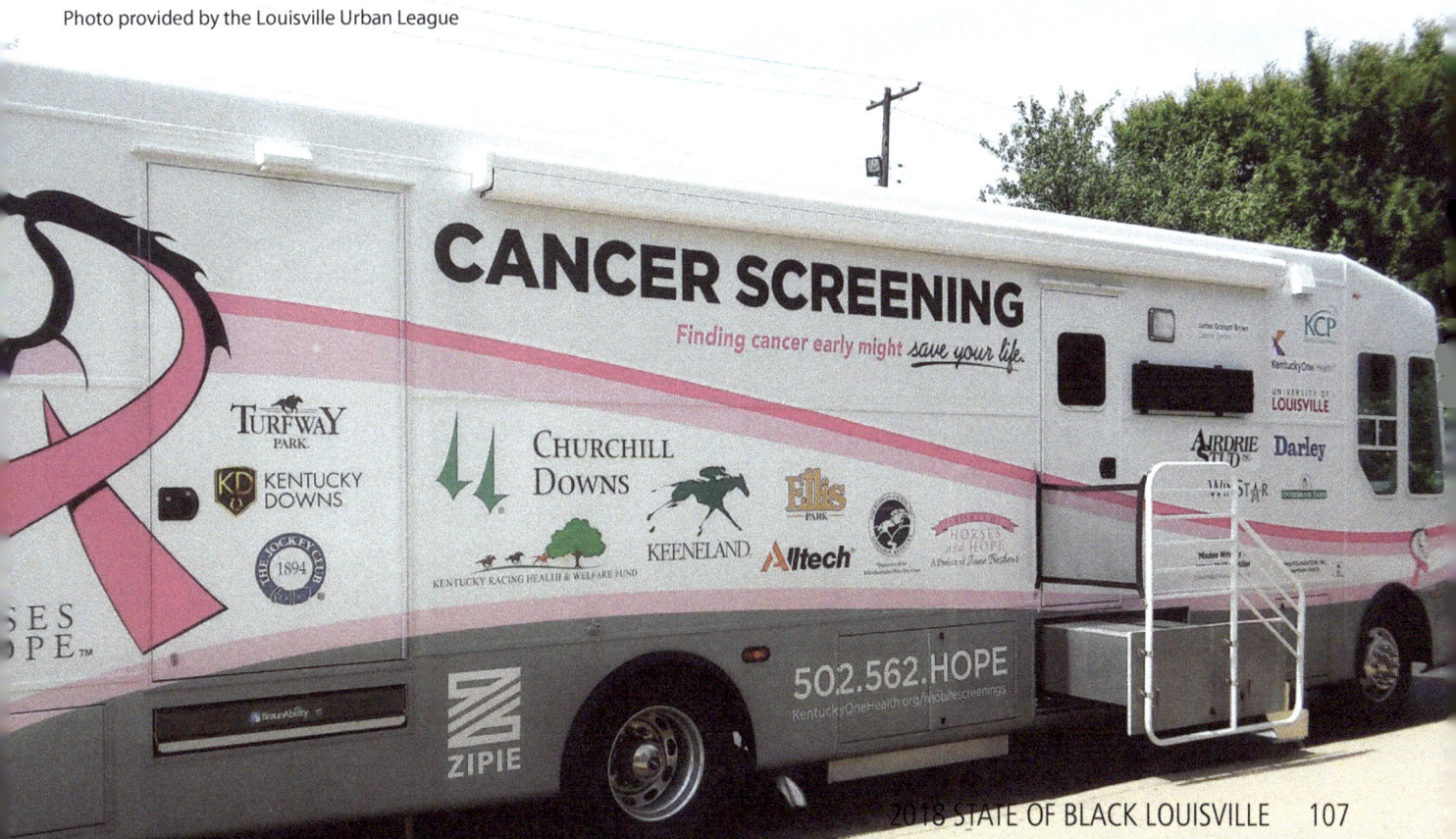

THE STATE OF FOOD JUSTICE IN BLACK LOUISVILLE: IS ACCESS TO FRESH FOOD A BASIC HUMAN RIGHT?

Karyn Moskowitz, Executive Director
Mary Montgomery, Uber Farmer Liaison
New Roots, Inc.

In 2007, Community Farm Alliance issued a report identifying the so-called "food deserts" of Louisville, much of which were in west Louisville and East Downtown.[138] The report speaks to the dearth of affordable fresh food to purchase in the neighborhoods, and the abundance of fast food restaurants and corner liquor stores. The authors connected the health inequity experienced by Black Louisvillians to fresh food inequality, including shorter life spans and higher rates of Type II diabetes and high blood pressure.

Not content to be classified strictly as a community with a deficit, leaders came together to formulate solutions. Unfortunately, the solutions failed to deliver results, including farmers' markets, mobile markets, resellers for local farmers, the Healthy in a Hurry Corner Store Initiative, and First Choice Market. Each of these initiatives came with their own set of challenges, but, for the most part, economics played a key role. Retail prices for fresh food, compared to

the price of processed and fast food, was simply too expensive. Many of these options were either sold, lost key leadership, lost key sponsorship/support, or simply ended up not being able to provide fresh food to the community in any significant amount as initially promised.

In 2009, with the resiliency that Kentuckians are known for, we picked ourselves up, dusted off our walking shoes, and hit the ground organizing around more sustainable solutions.

We knew that it was imperative that churches get involved, and that the movement for food justice had to be driven by those struggling with the challenges of food insecurity. We turned to the USDA "food desert" maps not to gaze into some purported emptiness as the name implies, but to identify leadership.

Out of this backdrop in June 2009, New Roots was

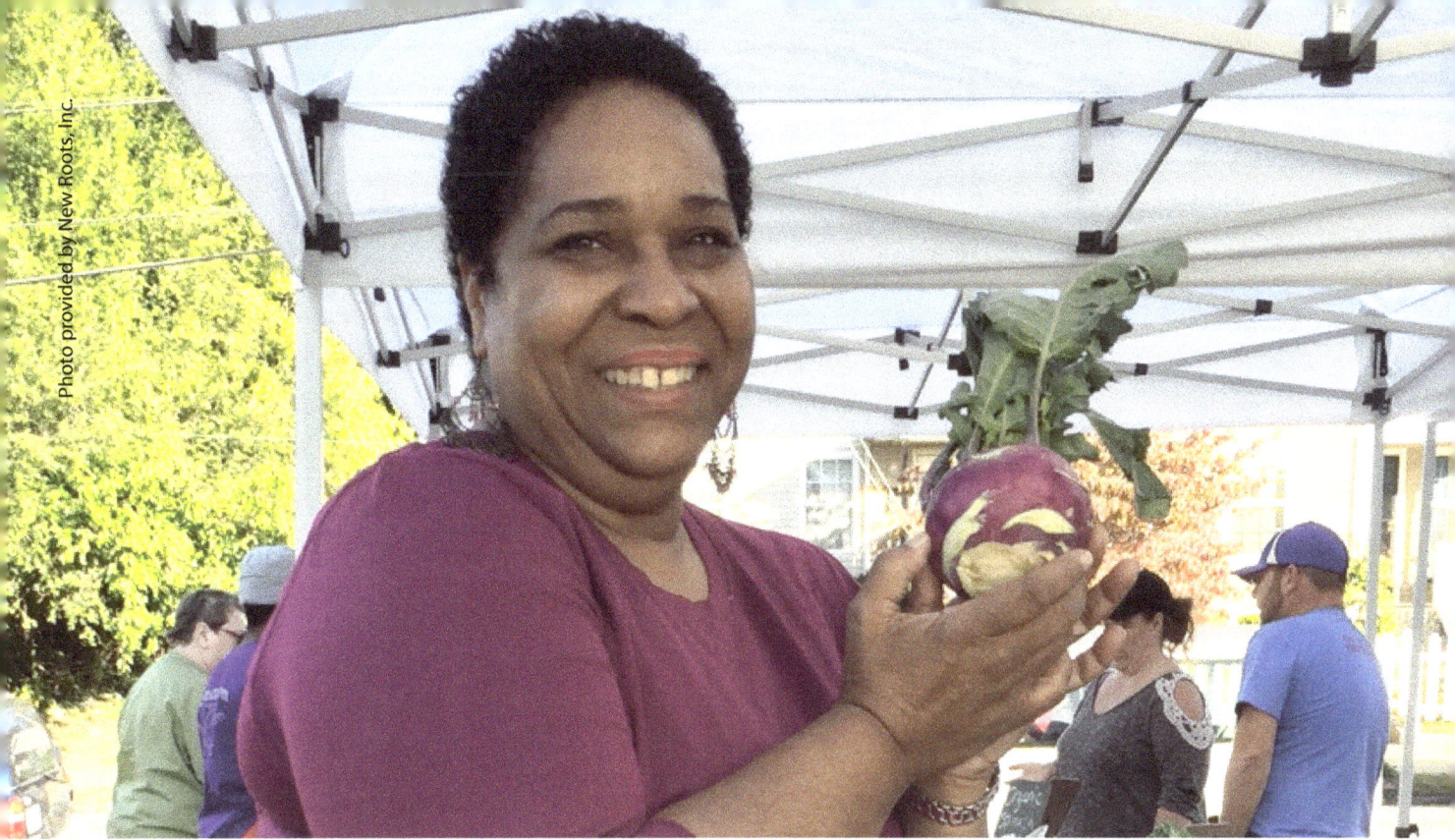

born and has continued to unite communities to spread food justice. Our tagline (created by Black Louisville) states, "Fresh food is a basic human right." We created a new model—utilizing grassroots community organizing —for fresh food access that is equitable and just. This Fresh Stop Market model grew out of both Black Louisville eaters and White rural farmers' feelings of isolation and abandonment by the industrial food system. We've united rural and urban Kentucky, Black and White Louisvillians, and other groups divided by historic redlining.

Fresh Stop Markets rely on families pooling their resources on an income-based sliding scale, ahead of the Markets, thereby guaranteeing orders and fair wages to farmers. The movement centers around the idea that everyone deserves access to the same local, organic food that can form the basis of a better quality of life. Black churches provide most of our leadership and host sites.

Fast forward to 2018, and we are happy to report that hundreds of volunteer leaders and "shareholders" continue to drive New Roots and the Fresh Stop

Markets with a passion that surprises many outside of this movement. This past year, we connected approximately 1,800 families (70% facing limited resources) to 50 Kentuckiana farmers to purchase 7,000 shares of local, organic, affordable, seasonal produce at our fourteen Markets. This coming season, we are growing to eighteen Markets.

Have we reached every family who struggles with fresh food insecurity? Is fresh food really a basic human right in Black Louisville and beyond? No. Our resources are limited, but we are busy fundraising to grow the movement. We have demonstrated that cooperative economics to combat fresh food insecurity in Black Louisville works today, just as it worked in years past when our ancestors pooled their resources to start their own benevolent societies.

We've shown that the statement "Black Louisville does not want to eat their vegetables" is just not accurate. We've formed community among people where it didn't exist before. We would love for all of Black Louisville to join us in building this movement.

THE IMPORTANCE OF VIOLENCE PREVENTION IN THE BLACK COMMUNITY OF LOUISVILLE

Yvette Gentry, Former Deputy Chief of Police of LMPD; Former Chief of Community Building for Louisville Metro Government

Last year, our community reached its highest homicide count in history. From January 1 to August 21, 2017, we lost 78 people to criminal homicide. At the same time, 162 people died from overdoses, largely caused by heroin and opioid use.[139]

Our reaction to the opioid epidemic has been to dedicate more resources to prevention and treatment for addiction. Our reaction to the high homicide rate has been mostly limited to increasing funding for public safety. I argue that we need to treat the public health crisis of violence with the same level of resources, respect, and commitment.

I approach this issue as a 27-year veteran of the largest police agency in Kentucky – Louisville Metro Police Department (LMPD) – including the role of Deputy Chief of Police. I also approach this issue as a public servant, having served as Chief of Community Building, and a mother of four wonderful and valuable Black boys who was also raised in this community myself.

Good policing is a critical component in violence reduction. Officer presence and engagement is significant to assisting community members regain the courage and comfort level to take back control of their public spaces that are being occupied by people promoting gang and drug activity. Police have been grappling with an unprecedented level of violence and a growing opioid epidemic, which has made it clear that *we cannot arrest our way out of these issues.* Communities that are making progress in reducing violent crime recognize and support the need to invest in more balanced approaches that focus on root causes.

Our country's incarceration rates have tripled over the last few decades[140] and rather than mitigating the problems in our communities, the removal of so

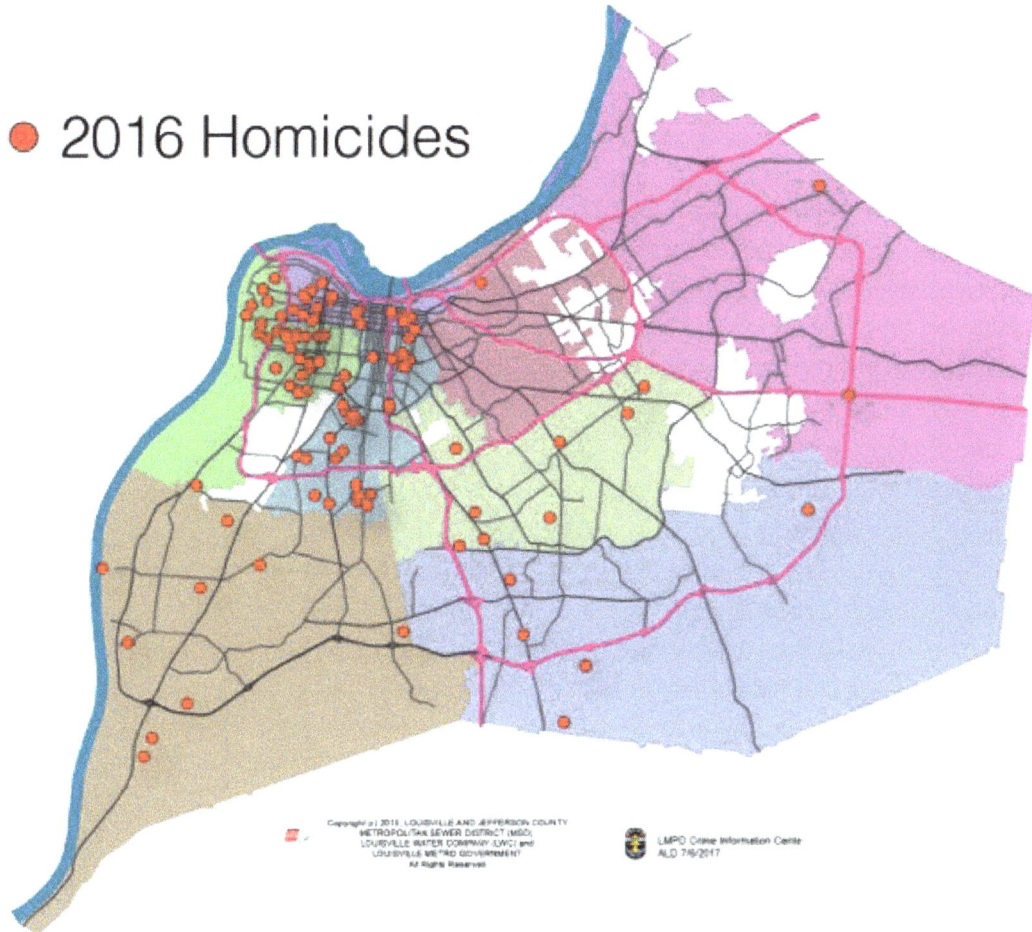

● 2016 Homicides

2017 Louisville Metro Police Department Crime Information Center

many Black men from the fabric of our community[141] [142] [143] has left us in a lurch, struggling to find a way forward.

In 2011, as the Assistant Chief of LMPD's Administrative Bureau, I was well resourced with a $143 million budget. As Chief of Community Building in 2017, however, I was not able to secure $143,000 in Louisville Metro Council's approved budget for grassroots organizations working in the areas we have collectively called "Zones of Hope." The irony and contrast in the numbers alone disturbed me greatly. I can accept that prevention strategies are not easily showcased to the community. But we can no longer tolerate them not being treated as the legitimate remedies for violence they are.

Violence and homicide is seen by many policy makers as an issue inherent to Black neighborhoods. It does not affect their daily lives because they are not integrated in those parts of the community. Of those 78 homicides, 55 (71%) are Black. Of the 162 overdose victims, 92% (149) are White.[144] There has been an earnest and cross-system response to the opioid crisis around the country. There has not been a sense of urgency to address the underlying and complex issues at the root of the violence in Black communities. Studies have been undertaken, but there is a disconnect when it comes to implementation. Dr. Michael McAfee, President of PolicyLink, alluded to this when he noted, "Leaders keep kicking the can down the road by participating in work-avoidance behaviors like discovering best practices, hosting conferences and webinars, writing reports, etc., without ever taking action to achieve results commensurate with the scale of the problem. If you are doing this, you are creating an unaccountable organization and colluding against transforming the lives of the children you are privileged to serve."[145]

No more discoveries are needed. No more research is required. We have every stat possible to support the fact that Black males are 5.5 times more likely to die of homicide than any other group in Louisville. We know that tools like Narcan will not cure addiction and the opioid crisis, but we fund them because it gives addicts a fighting chance until they receive a level of clarity to seek the help needed and gain the strength needed to take the needle from their arms or the pill from their mouths. We also know that there is no silver bullet, no one tool, to cure violence. The efforts to disrupt the cycle will give those caught in it an opportunity to change and help create hope for them until they have the clarity to put the guns down.

Let's get dedicated and require equitable funding from federal, state, and local levels for violence prevention. If we can give the same person three doses of Narcan a day at an average cost of $42 per dose,[146] then we can fund violence prevention offices and organizations at scale to produce change as it relates to gun violence.

Inequitable responses have helped create the conditions that plague many neighborhoods today. The drug epidemic of the 1980s and '90s devastated the Black community, leading to many vacant properties and one-person households. Our response was to approach this crisis simply as a moral and criminal vice, and it only exacerbated the problem. It was not handled with a public health lens. Now, we are still fighting to put a public health strategy in place for violence.

Do not be confused – this is a public health issue.

A multifaceted, systemic approach to solving the crisis of violence is needed and the first step is legislation. To aid in addiction prevention, the state was able to successfully push legislation that limited the number of opioids that a doctor can initially prescribe.[147] They are keenly aware of the need to limit the supply of drugs. The same strategic approach needs to be set forth beginning with limiting the guns that are so easy accessible to young people in urban environments.

At the same time, we need to focus on the systemic issues *we already know* leads to violence: lack of viable employment; disparate educational achievement levels; households broken up by the prison industrial complex; access to housing; and the ability to attain generational wealth.[148] [149] WE are holding these children every day and WE need to stand behind complex solutions to complex problems. The solutions to violence come by supporting legislation for violence prevention, by supporting politicians who dedicate resources to the prevention of violence, and by continuing to join in politics and public service to ensure our voices are heard.

In addition, the state needs to stop selling the weapons that officers confiscate back to the community at auction. If we aren't willing to destroy them, then hold them for a few years so we can evaluate the impact of that decision. We should do everything in our power to address these preventable deaths and the suffering that families endure. It has taken years for our broken systems to reach their stature, and it will take years to tear them down and build more equitable ones.

If you have the power to allocate, allocate more. If you are able to appropriate, appropriate more. If you are in a position to teach, give and advocate, double down on your efforts. If we believe we have more time to debate this issue, then it is obvious that we are not holding the same children.

GOOD MENTAL HEALTH: A PUBLIC HEALTH PRIORITY

Dr. Vicki P. Hines-Martin, Professor & Director
Office of Health Disparities and Community Engagement
School of Nursing, University of Louisville

Mental health in Black Louisville has not been discussed as a public health priority and, therefore, is not as clearly understood. It continues to be perceived negatively, sometimes as a personal failing, which adversely affects people who have experienced poor mental health. I use the term "emotional" rather than "mental" to highlight what is key: how you feel is intertwined with how you think and actions you choose as part of daily living. In addition, emotional health functioning has a physical basis not unlike other physical functioning, which can result in detrimental conditions like hypertension, diabetes, and cardiovascular disease.

The World Health Organization (WHO) identified in 2005 that "there is no health without mental health".[150] However, most are not aware that emotional health conditions as a group are considered the leading causes of disability, lost days of work, and suffering worldwide. Depression is ranked by the WHO as the single largest contributor to global disability among *all* health conditions; anxiety disorders are ranked 6th among all health conditions.[151]

Although poor emotional health can and does affect all types of people of all ages, research has clearly identified that the risk of poor emotional health outcomes is significantly increased by poverty (and its consequences related to poor or unstable housing, limited resources and education, and food insecurity); unemployment and underemployment; traumatic life events such as exposure to violence/abuse/neglect; social exclusion and racism; physical illness; and problems resulting from primary or secondary exposure to alcohol and drug use.

Most importantly, ongoing exposure to these social, environmental, and economic pressures results in toxic stress on the mind and body, which accumulates over time and adversely affects individual development and functioning as well as the functioning of families and ultimately the communities in which they live.[152] This effect is most important in the development of children and can have a life-long impact.

So what does this have to do with Black lives in Louisville? As you read the essays within this report, you'll see that many Black residents have greater disparity in educational attainment, annual income, higher incidences of chronic illness, and greater exposure to traumatic events such as violence and racism. Racism may be experienced from institutional structures or through micro-aggressions from others. It has been an ongoing, open discussion by the Black community and others in Louisville, and has increased during our current political climate. Each of these factors has significant association with higher risk for negative emotional health impact and *must* be considered as part of a genuine public health priority in Louisville.

Emotional health is not just the absence of emotional illness; it is "a state of well-being in which the individual realizes his or her own abilities, can cope with the normal stresses of life, can work productively and fruitfully, and is able to make a contribution to his or her community".[i] Therefore, recommendations for change in how we support the ability to accomplish and maintain this state of wellbeing in the Black community must include a multi-organizational, multi-focal approach that contains these key elements:

- ▶ We must partner with Black communities to best identify their priorities and struggles, and how these impact their emotional well-being.

- ▶ Refocus efforts for increased emphasis on emotional well-being support strategies that are culturally and socially tailored and concentrate on the strengths of Black communities using what is learned through collaboration with those community members. The greatest health benefit and the best use of precious resources comes from prevention rather than cure with any health condition.

- ▶ Implement prevention and early interventions strategies founded on an understanding that negative social, economic, and political factors do result in poor emotional health outcomes and that these must also be addressed to make a difference.

- ▶ Within the reality of limited resources, care of people already affected by emotional health disorders requires thoughtful application of available resources and resource development. This should be informed by accurate data about the population to be served, knowledge about best practice with diverse populations, and collaboration with Black communities through engagement to make health changes that are sustainable and acceptable to individuals being served.[153]

Louisville has much work to do in each of these areas to enhance the lives of Black Louisville.

GROWING UP BLACK IN LOUISVILLE

LaGraica Williams
Iroquois High School

I'm a 17-year-old, African American female who lives in Louisville, Kentucky. I am also a senior at Iroquois High School. I've faced many challenges, including trying to prove that just because I go to a school in a bad area of town that's also one of the schools with the lowest testing scores, that doesn't make me who I am today. I have also tried proving to my teachers that just because of my background, I haven't given up on myself, which is what I think they sometimes get from most kids in school.

I've dealt with teachers not pushing me to work my hardest when I was slipping off, seeming to not care if I was capable of more. One of my teachers once said, "There's no point in pushing the kids to do their best or to give more because they just don't care." That made me remind myself every day that no matter how hard it gets or how many times I get off track, I had to keep trying and I had to get back on top of things.

The classes are so big and the kids are so distracting. Many of them don't seem to care, which may cause the teachers to give up on the class as a whole. When you do ask for help after class, they tell you that you should've been paying attention. Yet, it's so hard to pay attention when you have kids throwing things and yelling at each other and arguing with the teacher. You'd probably say, "Why don't they send them to in-school suspension or call the parents?" That appears to have stopped working in elementary school. The parents come across as if they have stopped caring, or the kids just seem to be out of their control.

I live in the West End of Louisville. My school is located in south Louisville. Both are very similar, with liquor stores on every corner, abandoned houses down every street, and roads with piles of litter on the corner. You also can't walk two blocks without seeing a homeless person or someone who appears to be high on some type of drug. The nearest food market isn't really a food market; it's a convenient store. When we do visit a food market, it's filled with low-graded meat and rotted vegetables and fruits. If they are any good, they're out of our price range.

It's worth going out of our neighborhoods, at times, for fresh and better food. The experience is much different in the St. Matthews area or even the Jeffersontown area of the city, where I traveled to during my middle school years. Coming all the way from the West End, I had to wake up at five in the morning to get on the school bus and make that trip. The schools in my area either aren't the schools I'm assigned to or I didn't have the grades and accomplishments I needed at the time to get into those schools.

Being an African American in Louisville, this is what it's like for me. This is what I've lived with for the last 17 years. Everybody's view isn't the same; some Blacks have it better than others. However, that's not the case for me. I know our people deserve better.

WE ALL DESERVE COMMUNITIES THAT ARE SAFE, HEALTHY, AND HOPEFUL: ADDRESSING THE ROOTS CAUSES OF COMMUNITY VIOLENCE

Anthony Smith, Executive Director
Cities United

If we are really serious about making sure all Black children in Louisville grow up in communities that are safe, healthy, and hopeful, then we must confront our past, have honest conversations about our shortcomings, and be willing to make deep investments in our children and their families. It starts with believing that all our children and their families deserve stable housing, access to quality education, an economic system that supports new business development and a livable wage, and a more just criminal justice system.

Homicides touch all corners of Louisville, but those living in and around some neighborhoods in the West End of Louisville are the most affected by this form of community violence.

On July 6, 2017, Louisville Mayor shared his vision on how to capture the spirit of Muhammad Ali at the Muhammad Ali Center during his "Capturing Ali's

Spirit: Creating a City of Peace and Safety" event.[154] Race, zip code and lack of access to resources for safety, education, and career advancement make it nearly impossible to achieve the American dream. This has been the reality for too many of our families, for far too long. Maybe now that we are being honest about these facts, we will create some clear pathways forward. These pathways must be rooted in the communities that Black folks have traditionally called home and raised their families. They must be supported by strong programs and effective policies so that they are sustained and have a greater impact.

Below is a list of policies, programs, and organizations that we need to support and hold accountable if we are going to create pathways to promise for all of our children and address the root causes of community violence in our neighborhoods:

Louisville Homicides 1970–2016

1971 110

2016 117

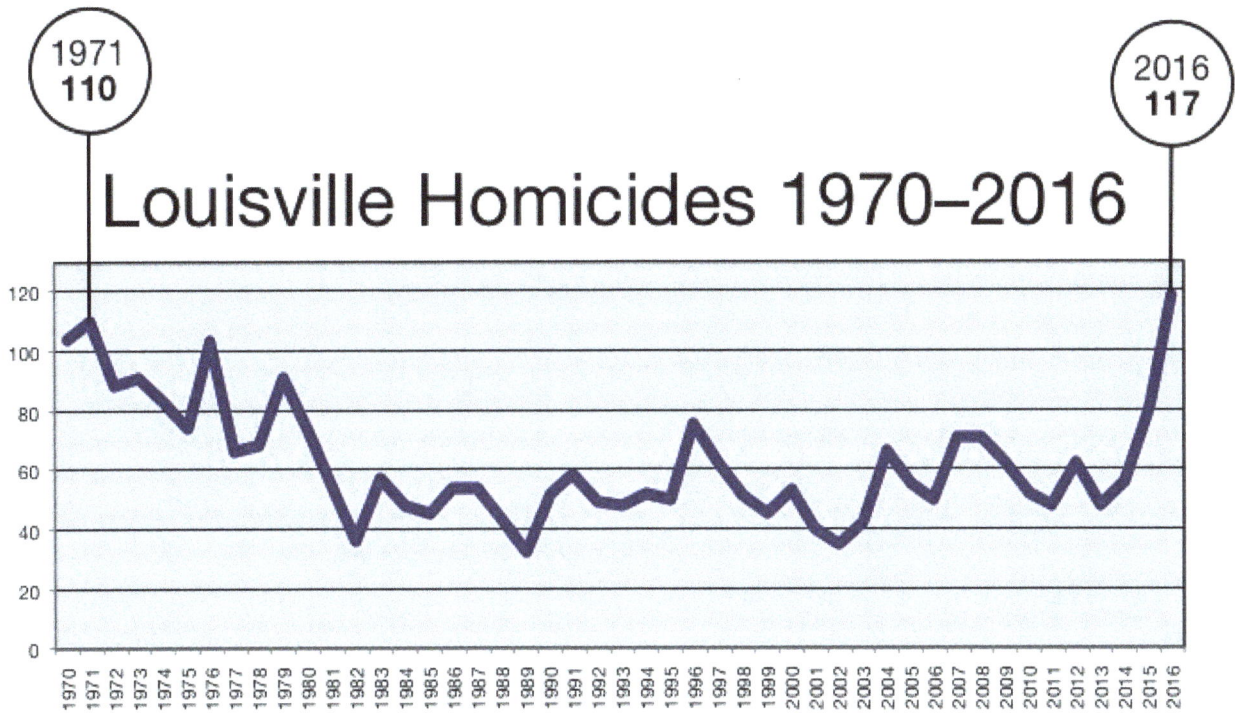

Credit: City of Louisville, Kentucky

PATHWAYS THAT SECURE SAFE, AFFORDABLE, AND STABLE HOUSING FOR ALL OUR FAMILIES

▶ The Louisville Metro Affordable Housing Trust Fund (LAHTF) was created by the Louisville Metro Council as a way for Louisville to invest additional local public funds to address the affordable housing shortage. Now that the mayor and council have committed nearly $10 million of the city's budget to support LAHTF,[155] it's our responsibility to make sure these funds are distributed equitable. We can do this by attending Metro Council meetings to show our support for LAHTF and ask questions about how the funds are being dispersed.

▶ Support organizations and programs that are working, by donating your time and dollars so that they can have the capacity to meet the demand: REBOUND, Inc.; Habitat for Humanity; and Jesus and A Job

PATHWAYS THAT MAKE SURE OUR CHILDREN ARE RECEIVING A HIGH-QUALITY K-12 EDUCATION AND ARE PREPARED TO SUCCEED IN COLLEGE

▶ JCPS Board of Education makes decisions every day that have critical impacts on our children's educational outcomes. We can no longer allow our voices and concerns to go unheard. Parents and community members must attend school board meetings, serve on the School-Based Decision Making Councils, and support the PTA. If we truly believe that education is the great equalizer, then we all need to do a better job at making sure all our children receive a quality education.

▶ Charter Schools. No matter your take on charter schools, they will be our reality starting as early as the 2018-2019 school year. With that in mind, we need to get ahead of the game by attending the planning meetings, research which models have worked for our children, and develop an agenda.

- 15,000 Degrees. Some of our Black leaders have committed to increasing the number of two- and four-year degrees in the Black community by 15,000 by the year 2020. For this to be a reality, we must build stronger support systems that look beyond getting students to college, but through college. This means students should have access to a computer and Wi-Fi, quality childcare, affordable transportation, and basic dorm room supplies. Not having these little things can prevent a student from being successful.

PATHWAYS TO ECONOMIC DEVELOPMENT AND GROWTH THAT INCLUDES NEW BLACK-OWNED BUSINESSES AND EMPLOYMENT WITH LIVABLE WAGE THAT CAN SUPPORT A FAMILY

- OneWest, which was created to establish new pathways to private and public capital in an effort to generate sustainable economic development and revitalization in West Louisville.

- The Nia Center was designed with a purpose of empowering people to develop a more meaningful life for themselves and their business.

- Louisville Urban League's Center for Workforce Development is a resource for individuals who are actively involved in job search, seeking a career change, or need job training.

PATHWAYS TO A JUST CRIMINAL JUSTICE SYSTEM

- Senate Bill 200. Passed in 2014, SB 200 is a comprehensive bill focused on improving the outcomes of our youth who are disproportionately affected by the criminal justice system.

- Senate Bill 120. Passed in 2017, this bill is designed to help people with criminal records stay out of jail and get back to work. It will save taxpayers and increase public safety by easing the transition back into society for those who have made mistakes.

- Police Reform. The Louisville Metro Police Department has adopted former U.S. President Barack Obama's 21st Century Policing recommendations. These recommendations could improve community relations within our neighborhoods and decrease our negative interactions with police officers.

Every child deserves to grow up in communities that are safe, healthy, and hopeful. The work we are doing, coupled with these recommendations, will aid in that.

URBAN LEAGUE, HUMANA CREATE 'IT STARTS WITH ME!'

Sadiqa N. Reynolds, President and CEO
Louisville Urban League
Virginia Kelly Judd, Former Executive Director
The Humana Foundation

"Hope has two beautiful daughters. Their names are anger and courage; anger at the way things are, and courage to see that they do not remain the way they are." – St. Augustine

The realities of health and health disparities in this city are stark and significant. If you live in west Louisville or Smoketown, the chances of developing a chronic illness such as diabetes or heart disease are higher. The chances of dying from certain cancers are higher. In fact, if you live here, on average you will die as much as 13 years sooner than the average person in other parts of Louisville. These realities are not of one's own choosing, but a birthright by virtue of zip code. The facts are frightening, unforgiving, and unfortunately not surprising.

We know that health is not simply a question of who is or is not "sick." It is more complicated than what you eat, how often you exercise, or who your doctor is. Rather, health is a combination of many factors that contribute to one's overall sense of well-being. The facts above are predictable because unemployment and underemployment are also higher in west Louisville. Educational attainment and environmental pollution are worse here, and the ability to access healthy, affordable foods and healthy activities is choked here.

All these things impact who is likely to become sick and how likely they are to stay that way. Many of these inequities are historical, systematic, and were created through policy. Thus, it will ultimately take policy to remedy and eradicate these issues.

As we work toward policy changes that will move the

needle, we must also work with partners to impact where we can, as much as we can, for as long as we can. Working together, we can change outcomes. That is why it is such an honor to stand together and announce the $225,000 Humana Foundation grant to the Louisville Urban League for "It starts with me!", our new community health initiative.

"It starts with me!" will attempt to tackle health disparities on a size and scale that the League has not tried before and that can't be done without alliances with community stakeholders. Teams of trained community health workers will attempt to reach families living in the Russell, California, Parkland, and Shawnee neighborhoods — our four west Louisville Zones of Hope. We are starting with the Zones of Hope, a place-based violence reduction strategy supported by the James Graham Brown Foundation, because we know the Zones have critical needs and we have an infrastructure in place, connecting individuals to jobs and educational opportunities.

The program will reach out to households, connecting with individuals and families to conduct health assessments and link them to partners like the Russell Walks Initiative, the Louisville Sports Commission, Leadership Louisville's Bingham Fellows,

New Roots, the Center for Mental Health Disparities at the University of Louisville, Gilda's Club, and many more.

We are not seeking to be a provider of any particular medical service or program, but we hope to play the role of connector, helping to tie individuals and families to resources already in existence and guiding them through obstacles and over any barriers to success. Our focus is on behavioral and social change. Our goals, like the issues we're facing, are not simple and they will not be easy to achieve.

The Louisville Urban League has been about the work of jobs, justice, education, and housing for almost 100 years. Now, with the help of the Humana Foundation, the League can firmly add health to that list.

We push you to find your courage. Join us in this fight for a healthier, more equitable Louisville. Or take up your own particular cause. Just don't allow anger to go unchecked. For it is only through our courage to face the things that anger us that our hope might be realized.

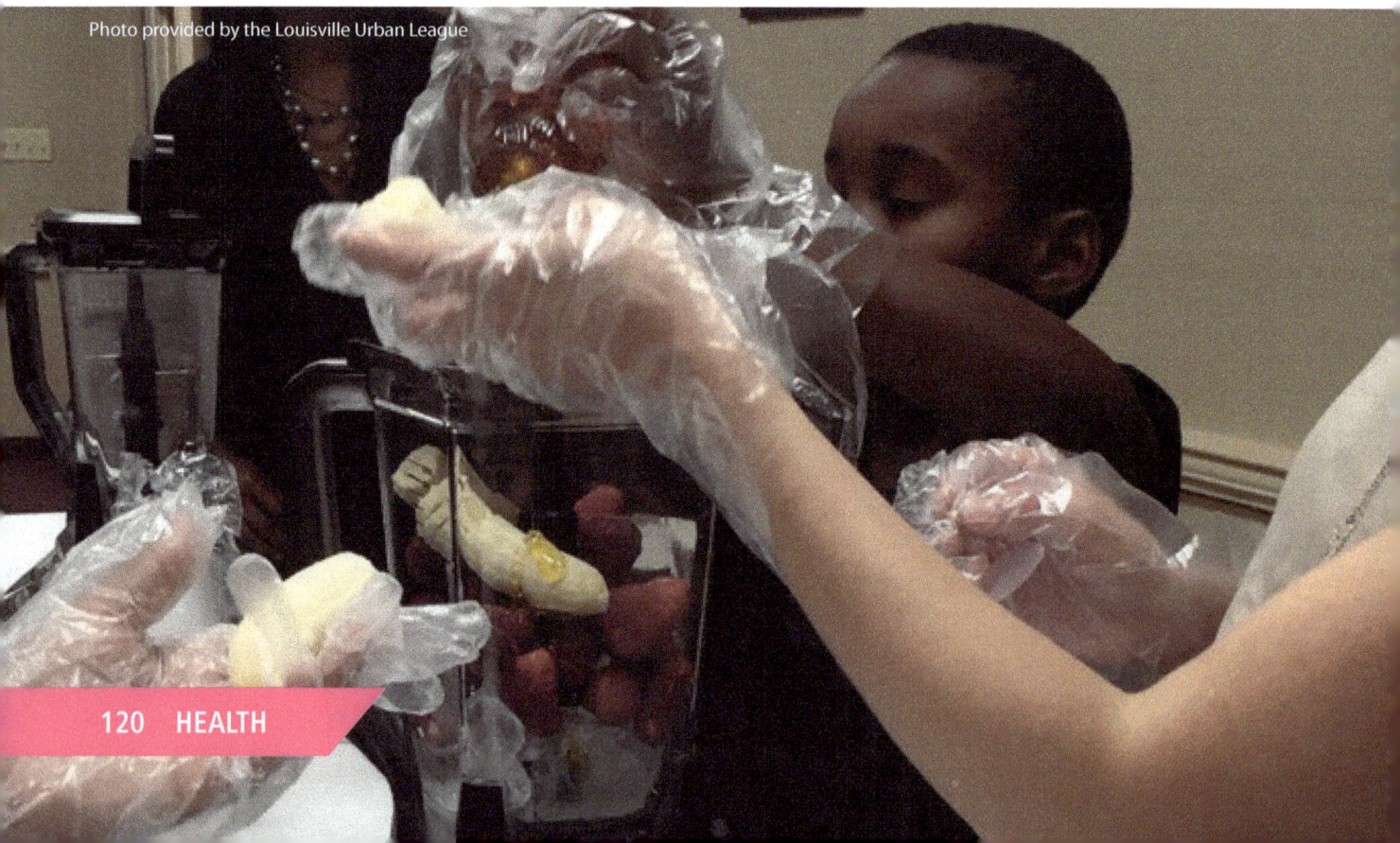

Photo provided by the Louisville Urban League

FATHERHOOD IN BLACK LOUISVILLE: CHALLENGES AND RESOURCES IMPACTING PATERNAL INVOLVEMENT

Dr. Armon R. Perry, Associate Professor
Kent School of Social Work, University of Louisville

Family is the primary institution in society. As such, it impacts and is impacted by all other community institutions. Given that contemporary society has raised the bar by adding commitments to nurturing and caregiving to the traditional role of breadwinner, earning the title of "good father" is more difficult than ever before.

For Black fathers in Louisville, this means that they must find ways to effectively navigate several micro and macro systems. In other words, Black fathers in Louisville are charged with taking financial responsibility for their children while also taking more active roles in their lives. This is happening concurrently with shifts in several of the institutions that have historically facilitated men's roles within families.

Table 1 displays 2016 U.S. Census Bureau (retrieved from the 2015 American Community Survey) data indicating that in Jefferson County, Kentucky, less than one-third of Black males over the age of 15 (e.g. 30.1% of Black men) are married.[156] Moreover, only 15.9% of the Black men reported having earned at least a bachelor's degree and 40.7% of Black men ages 16-64 were either unemployed or not in the labor force.

Although no data on cohabitation were available, the demographic data that were available indicate that only 38.5% of Louisville's Black families were married couples and 85.3% of single-parent households were headed by females with no husband. Keep in mind the Census Bureau defines family as, "a group of two people or more (one of whom is the householder) related by birth, marriage, or adoption and residing together."

While living away from one's children does not always mean being an uninvolved father, non-resident status does place one at risk for disengagement.[157] Taken together, these data begin to explain that most

TABLE 1. BLACK MALE DEMOGRAPHICS JEFFERSON COUNTY, KENTUCKY

Variable	Category	Sub-Category	Frequency
Black Households	Family Household	Non-family Households	22,362
		Married Couple Family	14,024
		Total	36,386
	Other Households	Female headed, no husband	18,857
		Male headed, no wife	3,260
		Total	22,117
Marriage Rates	Black Males	Never Married	27,956
		Married	16,460
		Separated	1,786
		Widowed	1,143
		Divorced	7,362
		Total	54,707
Income	Black Male	Median	24,030
Employment	Black Males 16-64	Employed	28,356
		Unemployed	6,080
		Not in Labor Force	13,443
		Armed Forces	75
		Total	47,954
Education	Black Males 25 and Up	Less than HS Diploma	6,231
		HS Diploma or GED	15,806
		Some College	13,687
		BS or more	6,743
		Total	42,467

of Louisville's Black families do not represent the traditional, married, two-parent nuclear family form that is often held up by the larger society as optimal. Moreover, despite the fact that Black families have always embraced alternative family forms to buffer themselves from the deleterious effects of poverty, patriarchal and hegemonic conceptualizations of masculinity and fatherhood persist.

These notions are manifested and reinforced through policy and media in Louisville. Examples include publishing an annual list of "deadbeat parents" and airing a local television show in which child support delinquent parents (disproportionately Black fathers) have their family matters adjudicated and broadcast over local airways and the internet.

In sum, the combination of relatively low marriage rates, high unemployment and underemployment rates, and low educational attainment means that many of Louisville's Black fathers are in precarious positions with regard to their continued access to and involvement with their children.

LOCAL RESOURCES

Although Black fathers in Louisville face many challenges, they also have access to a number of government, private non-profit, and grassroots initiatives designed to support them in their efforts to be engaged fathers. These initiatives include the work of Healthy Babies Louisville (HBL), 502 Fathers, 2NOT1, Brothers Helping Brothers, the 4 Your Child fatherhood program, and Jefferson County Public Schools (JCPS).

Administered by the Louisville Metro Department of Public Health and Wellness, HBL coordinates father friendliness training and technical support for local organizations interested in increasing men's participation in human and social services. Public Health and Wellness' Healthy Start program also offers 502 Fathers, an initiative that provides fatherhood-specific parent education workshops to men with infants and a social media campaign aimed at raising awareness about the importance of fathers.

2NOT1 is a local non-profit organization founded by local practitioner Shawn Gardner. 2NOT1 aims to influence both the larger culture around fatherhood, as well as the individual behavior of the fathers it serves. In so doing, it strives to "make fatherhood normal" by providing services including Teen Fathers University, a parenting skill intervention that targets teenage and young adult fathers, mothers' forums designed to encourage co-parenting, and an annual Fathers' Day Picnic.

Brothers Helping Brothers (BHB) is a grassroots initiative organized by local businessman and community activist Jerald Muhammad. BHB is a group-based, self-help cohort offering support to a cross section of Black men who are committed to self-reflection, personal improvement, and accountability. The culture of the meetings is informal and non-judgmental, making it a safe space for the men to share failures and celebrate victories all

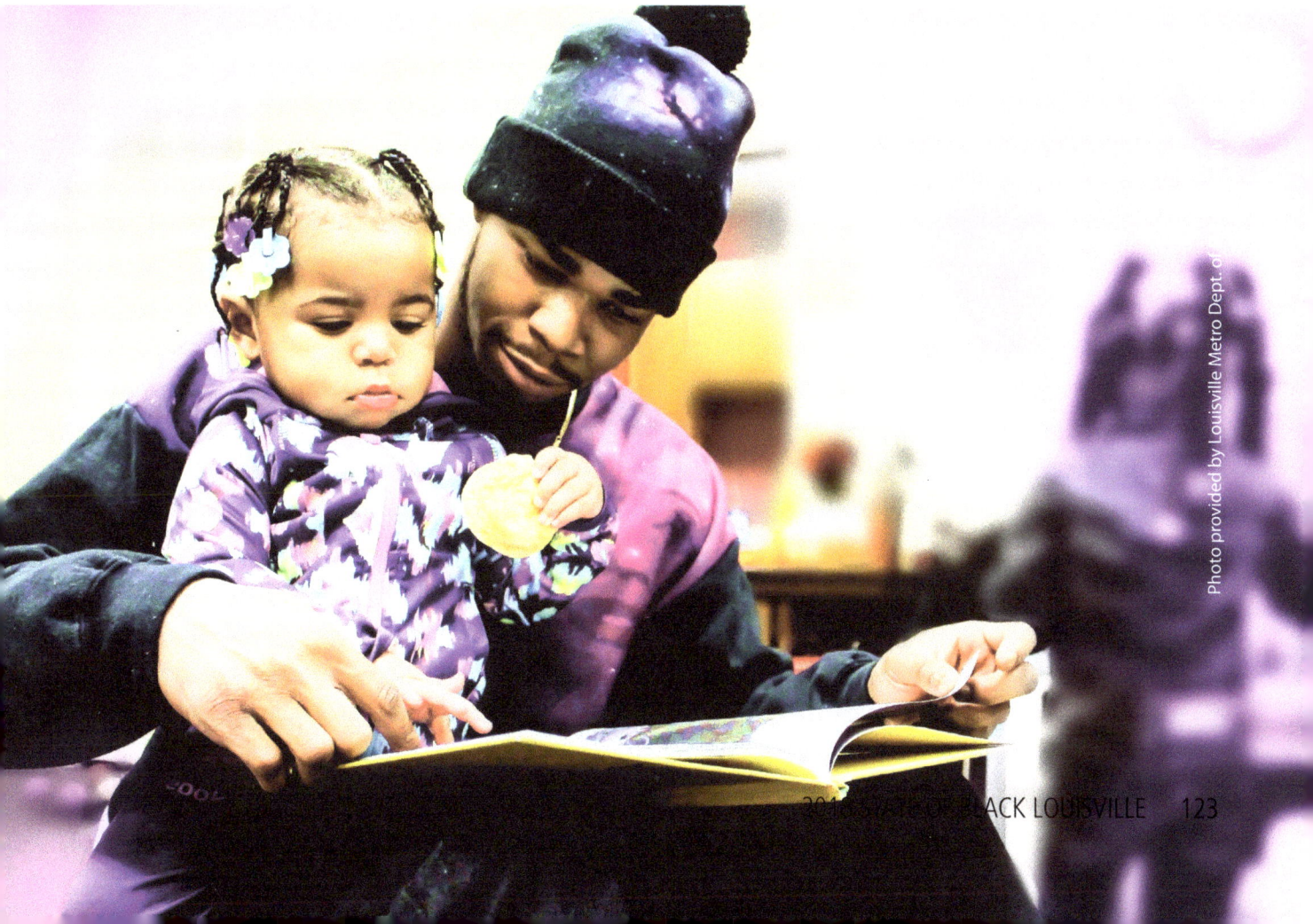

Photo provided by Louisville Metro Dept. of

while building a sense of community with men who understand the unique challenges associated with being a Black father in Louisville.

Directed by myself, the University of Louisville's Kent School of Social Work implements the 4 Your Child fatherhood program. This federally funded grant project enrolls non-resident fathers into a program featuring 28 hours of fatherhood-specific parent education and up to six months of case management services. The program and its rigorous evaluation are designed to serve as a model for bridging the gap between fatherhood practitioners and researchers.

Jefferson County Public Schools (JCPS) is involved in promoting fatherhood through its Head Start Male Initiative. The Head Start Male Initiative leverages relationships with local parents and professionals to ensure that children have access to positive male role models during their preschool years. Similarly, several JCPS schools have WATCH DOGS chapters. WATCH DOGS are informal programs that create volunteer opportunities for fathers to emphasize the important role that they play in encouraging social and emotional development, as well as academic achievement.

POLICY RECOMMENDATIONS

Many concerns about fathers' involvement with their children are born out of policy changes and macroeconomic trends leading to cultural shifts away from the traditional, married, two-parent nuclear family form. Therefore, it stands to reason that any effective response would include policy prescriptions.

First, policymakers should be encouraged to support proposals to eliminate the gender gap (*i.e.* discrepancies between the pay that men and women earn for doing similar work). History tells us that social science and the broader society first began to pay attention to fathers' involvement in the 1970s when large numbers of women entered the paid labor force. [158] We also know that despite their gender role orientations and aspirations for being

involved fathers, many men increase their work hours after the birth of a child due to real or perceived pressures to provide financially. [159] Thus, promoting gender equality in pay would simultaneously decrease the breadwinning pressure that many men feel, while also providing women with an incentive to pursue or maintain their careers after the birth of a child rather than both defaulting to socially prescribed and rigidly defined gender roles.

Second, policymakers should be encouraged to support proposals for paid parental leave with designated portions reserved exclusively for fathers. For decades, many European countries have made provisions for parents to take job-protected, compensated leave following the birth of a child. Moreover, in several of these countries (*e.g.* Italy, Finland, and Slovenia), there is also policy specifying paternity leave as a way to encourage fathers to engage in caregiving. [160]

Finally, more work should be done to change the culture around fatherhood. Healthy Babies Louisville, 502 Fathers, and 2NOT1 have already begun this awareness-raising work, but more is needed. This is important because it is not enough to simply create policy that encourages men to spend more time with their children. These initiatives need to be accompanied by work that aims to ensure that fathers are free to choose nurturing and caregiving without fear of stigma, ridicule, or sanction. By working to de-gender parenting and dismantling traditional, and in many cases, antiquated notions of fatherhood, practitioners, researchers, and advocates can help Louisville live up to its self-proclaimed moniker of Possibility City.

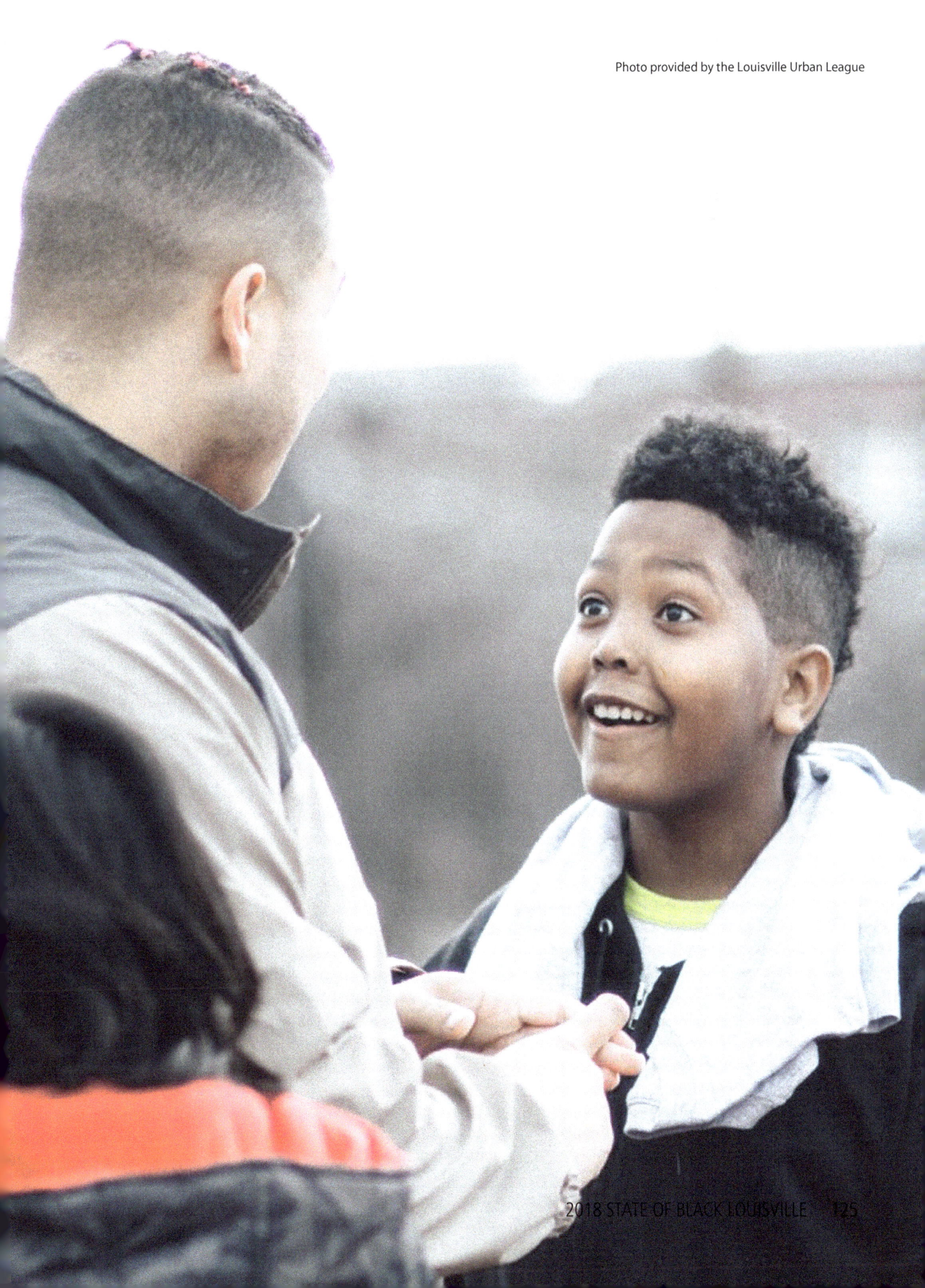

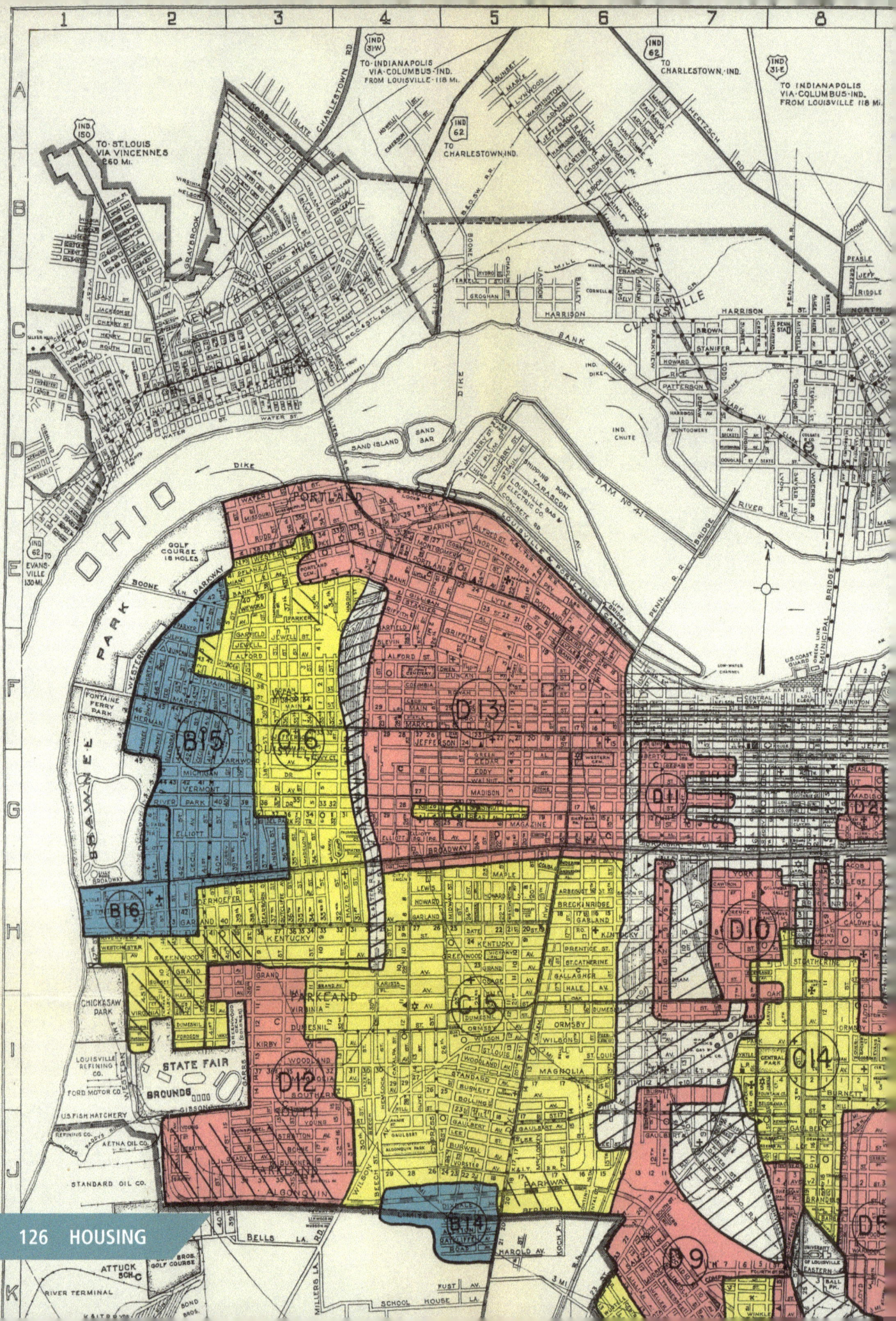

HOUSING

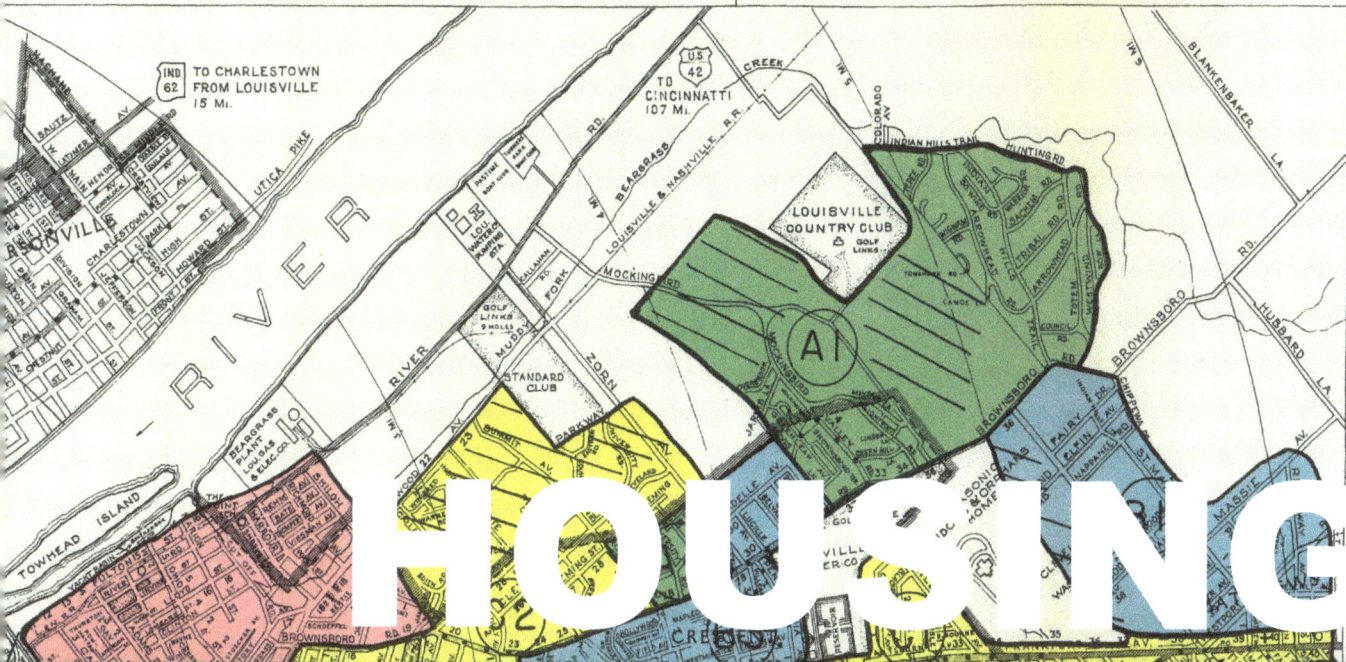

Today, 50 years after the Fair Housing Act of 1968, we still find ourselves, throughout the nation and here in Louisville and in Kentucky, working to ensure the furthering of fair housing.

The National Fair Housing Alliance recently released a report that noted people of color, persons with disabilities, and other marginalized groups continue to be unlawfully shut out of many neighborhoods.[161] Since the fall of 2016, there has been an uptick of hate crimes involving people who were harassed in their neighborhoods or at their apartments, university dormitories, or homes. Housing segregation continues from the deliberate discriminatory policies and practices by the federal government, the housing industry, and local communities.

The Kentucky Commission on Human Rights has witnessed an increase in housing discrimination over the past 10 years. In 2007, we investigated 30 housing complaints; in 2016 we investigated 74. For more than a hundred years, our city, state and nation have enacted laws, ordinances, and customs or practices which, either by design or impact, have served to damage, weaken, disrupt and generally destabilize African American communities all across America. Louisville and Kentucky are no exception. The sorted history of housing discrimination included redlining, restrictive covenants, discriminatory steering by real estate agents, and restricted access to private capital.

Government-sanctioned redlining, another form of institutional racism, started around 1934 and its lingering effects continue even today. Louisville, like many other cities in Kentucky, enacted

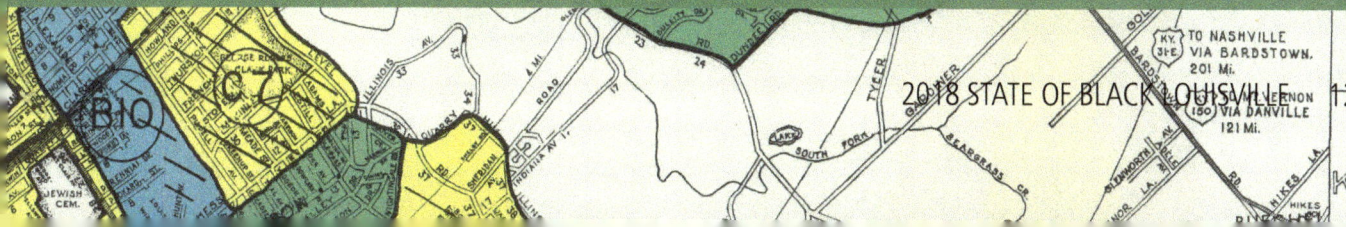

racially-biased ordinances, designed to keep Blacks from residing in predominantly White neighborhoods. In 1917, in the case of Buchanan v. Warley, which originated in Louisville, the U.S. Supreme Court struck down Louisville's racially-biased zoning ordinance as an unconstitutional interference by the city into the individual's right of contract. This did not stop housing segregation. Private restrictive covenants existed from 1920-1968.[162] These clauses were put into deeds to restrict Blacks and other minorities from purchasing the property. The Fair Housing Act declared these covenants illegal.

While that law was designed to provide equal housing opportunity, it also resulted in White flight, racist scare tactics, and blockbusting. Today, we find Louisville being the fourth-most residentially segregated city in the nation.[163] This segregation feeds directly into other social issues that disproportionately impact African American and other minority communities such as:

- ▶ Hate crimes
- ▶ Racial profiling
- ▶ Economic inequality
- ▶ Voter suppression and gerrymandering
- ▶ Educational achievement gaps

John J. Johnson, Executive Director
Kentucky Commission on Human Rights

- ▶ High school dropout rates
- ▶ Lack of equal quality education
- ▶ Inadequate health care
- ▶ Insufficient transportation…

… and many, many other issues too numerous to mention here.

To combat housing discrimination, aggressive fair housing public education campaigns, stronger regulations on lending practices, and more funding for affordable housing is necessary. We should strive not only to know and understand the history of housing discrimination in our city and state, but we must then seek to fully comprehend the depth and breadth of the damage and devastation that discriminatory practice has caused multiple generations of families.

In the area of housing, we must work to encourage desegregation of all Kentucky's cities through affirmatively furthering fair housing by supporting scattered-site, moderate, low-income housing throughout the commonwealth. Issues related to homelessness should also be a high priority for our city. During the 2016-17 school year, there were 5,765 homeless students in JCPS, of which 49.6% are African American.[164]

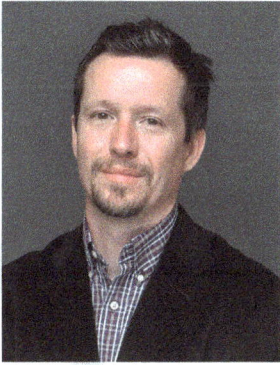
JOSHUA POE, Independent
Researcher

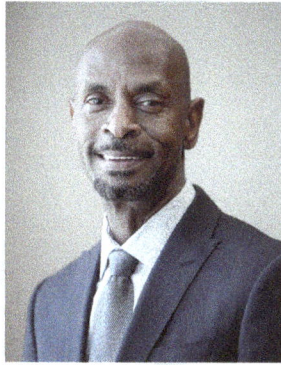
KEVIN DUNLAP, REBOUND, Inc.

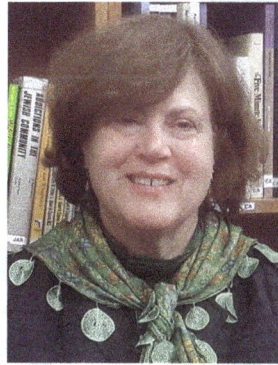
CATHY HINKO, Metropolitan Housing
Coalition

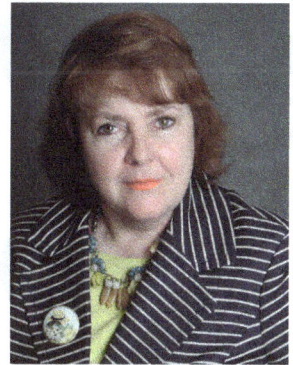
LISA THOMPSON, Louisville Urban
League

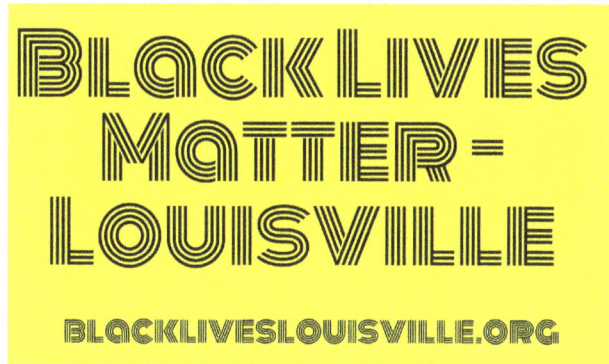

Black Lives Matter - Louisville

BLACKLIVESLOUISVILLE.ORG

CHANELLE HELM AND "SCZ", Black Lives Matter Louisville

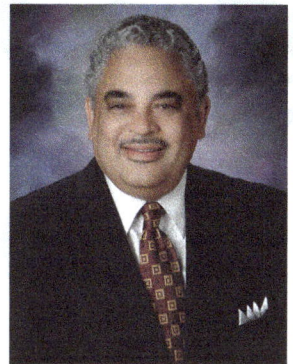
JOHN J. JOHNSON, Kentucky
Commission on Human Rights

REDLINING LOUISVILLE: THE RACIST ORIGINS OF CITY PLANNING AND REAL ESTATE

Joshua Poe, Independent Researcher and Activist

"Not everything that is faced can be changed, but nothing can be changed until it is faced." – James Baldwin

Author and journalist George R. Leighton visited Louisville in 1938, after which he opined in Harper's Magazine that the River City was a place that "paid great attention to food and drink, but for the rest, let well enough alone."[165]

That same year, local real estate interests colluded with the federal government to create a systematic form of residential apartheid that became known as redlining. The redlining maps created a rating system for property valuation and loan security to be used by private banks, but kept classified from the public. This system decided who would get home loans and who would not. The highest-graded areas were described as "homogenous," meaning "American businessman and professional men."[166] Neighborhoods with Black residents, or even those with the "threat of infiltration" by Black residents, were not considered "best" or "American." Black neighborhoods invariably received the lowest rating, eliminating their access to mortgage insurance, credit, wealth, and capital for decades.

Areas that were redlined in the 1930s show high correlations with current trends in poverty, segregation, crime, vacant properties, poor public health, mortgage denials, and a host of other categories. The rating system used "restrictions set up to protect neighborhoods" as a favorable factor in grading an area, meaning restrictions that prohibited the sale of property to Black people. The highest-ranked area in the 1938 maps were the neighborhoods of Mockingbird Valley, Rolling Fields, and Indian Hills (40207), not because they contained the highest property values or the nicest homes,

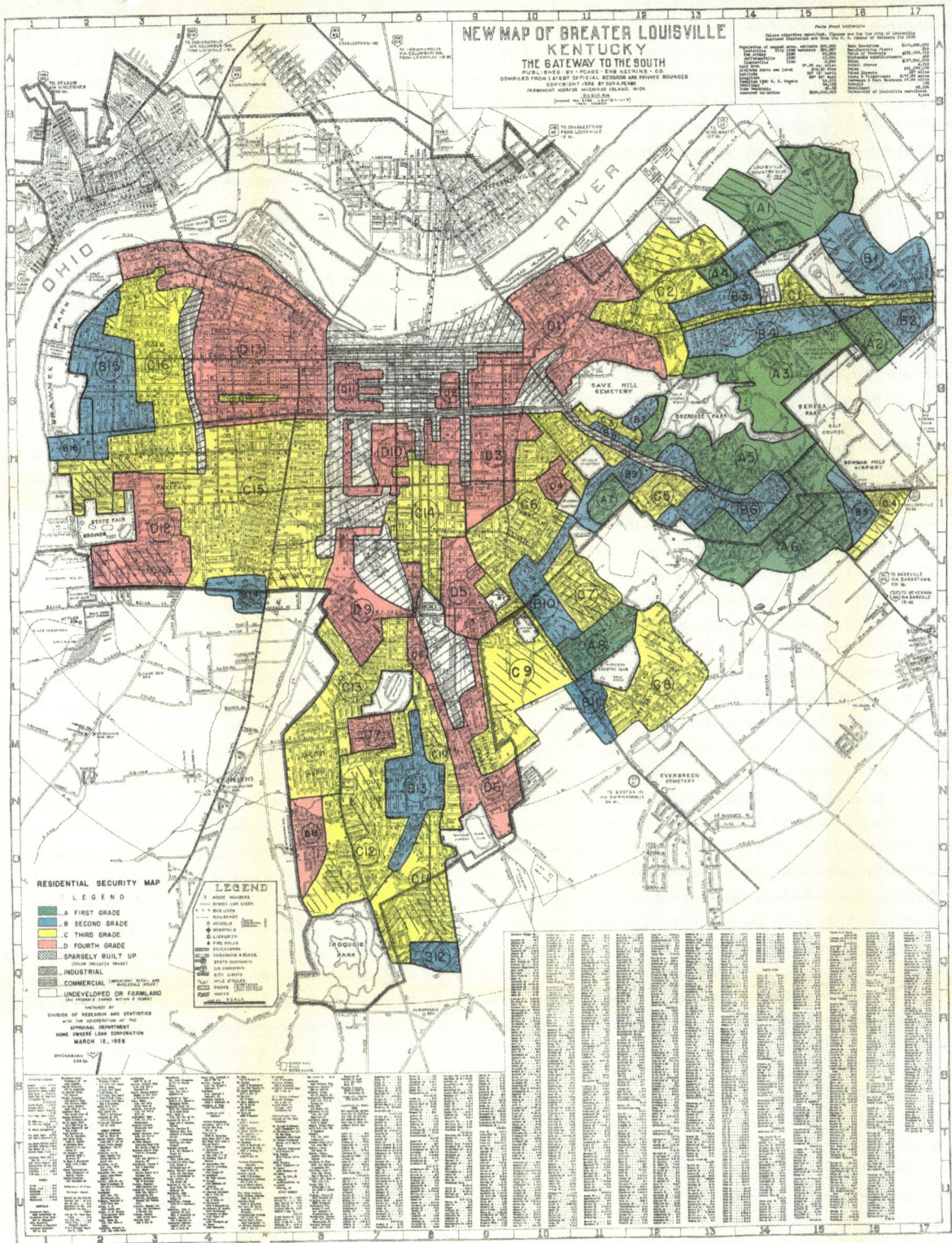

NEW MAP OF GREATER LOUISVILLE
KENTUCKY
THE GATEWAY TO THE SOUTH

The 1938 HOLC "security" map, which categorizes neighborhoods from "best" to "hazardous," is a striking visual document of the long history of racially-based housing discrimination. Four colors of the map dictated to lenders where they should and shouldn't lend. Areas shaded green were considered "first grade" and at the time were "synonymous with the areas where good mortgage lenders with available funds" lived or wanted to live, according to the 1938 explanation.

but because they were "one of the highest restricted areas" in the city. As the property values in these subdivisions have increased since 1938, so did the wealth accumulation of their residents.

That this wealth was created based on the exclusion of Blacks is one more insidious self-fulfilling prophecy of White supremacy. To this day, these neighborhoods have some of the highest average residential property values in the county and there was not one Black resident living in the area, according to the 2010 U.S. Census data.

In contrast, the east Russell neighborhood (40203) was described as the "worst area of the city," with a "low type of property and inhabitant." Although the boundaries are not a precise match today, Black population for the Russell neighborhood (Security Grade D Area 11) in 1938 was 80%.[167] Most recently, that percentage from the 2010 Census was 91.68%. Additionally, the Russell neighborhood today has the highest population density and the highest concentration of poverty in the region.[168] The census tract that encompasses east Russell has an annual median income of $8,707 and over 82% of the residents live below poverty level.

While redlining dictated the flow of capital in the city and created barriers for Blacks economically, the profession of city planning was created to segregate U.S. cities spatially.

In 1917, the U.S. Supreme Court abolished the practice of zoning based on race in the landmark Louisville case Buchanan v. Warely. This case helped shape and create the new profession of city planning, as planners became necessary to create subtler, de facto measures of ensuring racial segregation. Residential zoning, highway construction, and urban renewal were all employed to restrict Black residents to the least desirable areas of the city.

In the aftermath of the Warely case, Frederick Law Olmstead Jr., stated in 1918 that good zoning

policy had to be distinguished from "the legal and constitutional question," and that "in any housing developments which are to succeed…racial divisions…have to be taken into account."[169] [170] Famed planner Harlan Bartholomew said that the purpose of zoning was to prevent movement into "finer residential districts…by colored people."[171] He was responsible for highway placement in many cities and created the idea of industrial zoning next to Black neighborhoods, leading to long-term health consequences and environmental injustices for the Black community.

Bartholomew arrived in Louisville in the late 1920s to develop the city's first comprehensive plan. In 1932, he was tasked with devising a plan for the Russell neighborhood and published a document in response titled, "The Negro Housing Problem in Louisville," where he concluded: "There are a number of obstacles that are fundamental to any scheme for improving housing conditions among Negroes. [These include a] lack of desire among a large portion of the population for something better than they are accustomed to… If it were possible to create among the Negro masses a real desire for decent accommodations, the slums would automatically eliminate themselves."[172]

This document exposed the White supremacist ideology inherent in city planning and put in motion the forces that demolished larges sections of the Russell neighborhood. The purpose of early city planning was to segregate America; one of main purposes of city planning today is to gentrify neighborhoods, however unintentionally.

The accompanying image from 1932 shows Bartholomew's redesign plans for what became Beecher Terrace.[173] The design on the left is the traditional urban design that incorporates all the metrics currently used by urban planners to improve quality of life. The current efforts in Russell are eerily reminiscent of the past as planners from out of town descend on Louisville to bring this traditional urban

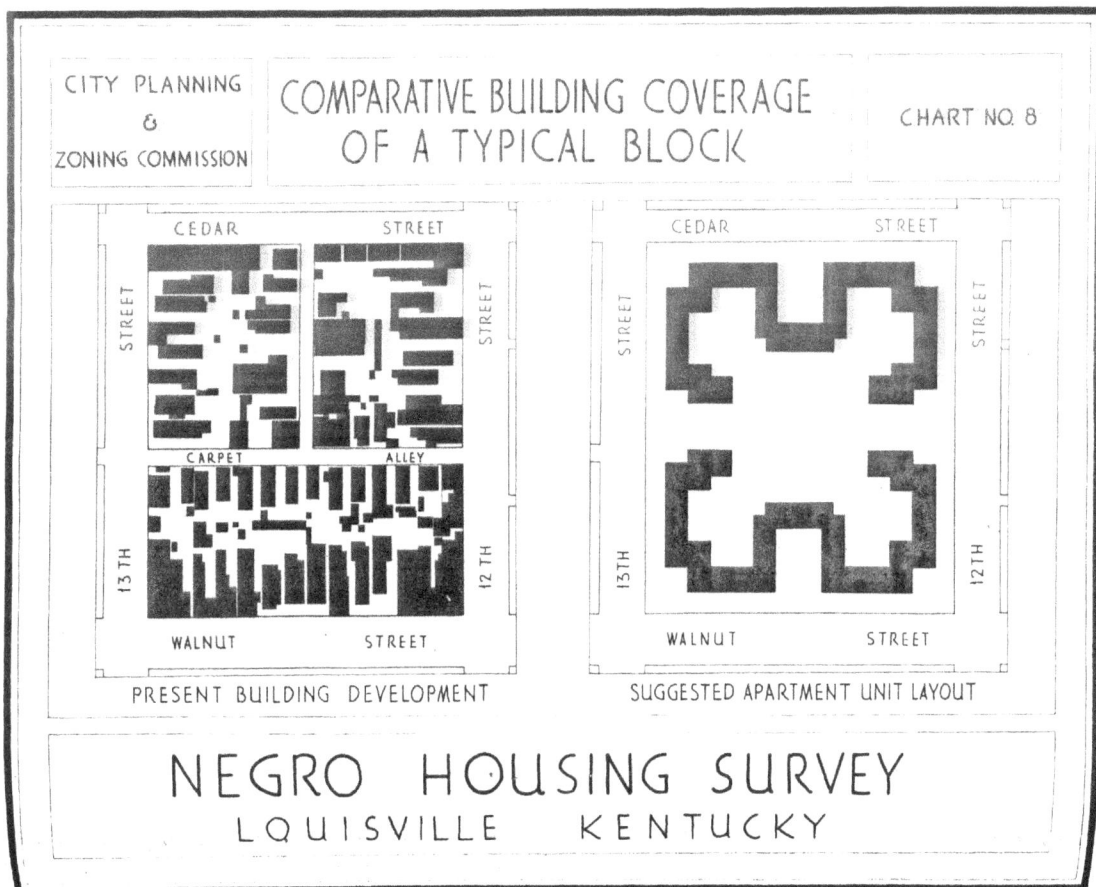

CITY PLANNING & ZONING COMMISSION

COMPARATIVE BUILDING COVERAGE OF A TYPICAL BLOCK

CHART NO. 8

CEDAR STREET

CARPET ALLEY

WALNUT STREET

PRESENT BUILDING DEVELOPMENT

CEDAR STREET

WALNUT STREET

SUGGESTED APARTMENT UNIT LAYOUT

NEGRO HOUSING SURVEY
LOUISVILLE KENTUCKY

typology back to the neighborhood.

But, while the traditional design will improve Russell, by the time it is implemented, the current residents will be gentrified and displaced by what city officials and planners call a "mixed income community" – a dog whistle term that means displacement of low-income residents by more affluent, White millennials.

While redlining devalued areas in west Louisville and confined Black residents to the West End, it also overvalued areas in the eastern section of the county, skewing any notion of a free market economy. This artificially-inflated market helped create a demand pattern of low-density sprawl that continues to accelerate today. New infrastructure investments in the east such as the new I-265 Lewis and Clark Bridge and Parklands of Floyd's Fork have facilitated new residential development outside the Gene Snyder loop at an unprecedented rate that is disproportionate to anything in the urban core.

Although redlining was determined illegal in 1972 through the Community Reinvestment Act, it became systematized in current real estate market analysis and the historic alliance between the public and private sector continues to determine the spatial allocation of real estate investment.

One way this alliance is operating in Louisville is through the Louisville Creating Affordable Residences for Economic Success (CARES) initiative, where housing advocates have partnered with local government and private developers to support building more multi-family housing far from west Louisville. The goal of the Louisville CARES program is "to address the need for affordable housing for low- to moderate-income, working households by establishing a revolving loan fund to create and retain affordable housing units over the next 30 years."[174]

The 2016 round of low-interests loans from the initiative have allocated over $5 million for 21 affordable housing units in Norton Commons and 216 units in southeastern Jefferson County, both developments outside I-265. In all, Louisville CARES has dedicated over $10 million to six projects as of October 2017; all but one are outside the I-264 beltway and none are within any former redlined areas or west Louisville.

Through efforts to desegregate the West End, housing advocates are supporting building affordable housing far outside the urban core, based on the belief that Black people will benefit from living in predominantly White neighborhoods. As Angela Davis warned in her visit to Louisville in November 2016, "Beware the call to integrate and assimilate. We have been told that the solution to racism was to integrate Black people into racist schools and racist places of employment… It is not a question of simply incorporating Black people or native people into a racist society. It is a question of transforming the very society that has produced racism and economic injustice. This is the work we need to accelerate right now."[175]

We see the systemic legacy of redlining in how current projects receive public funding. In September 2017, Louisville Metro Government announced its approval to support the Louisville Urban League in building a $30 million indoor track and field facility in the Russell neighborhood. However, there was no financing plan for the project. In contrast, a month later, the Louisville Metro Council voted to approve a $30 million bond for a $200 million professional soccer stadium in Butchertown after only two council meetings.

The pace of approval and financing these projects highlights the discrepancies in how capital moves in White, gentrifying areas east of downtown versus predominantly Black neighborhoods west of downtown. Certainly, there are other factors involved in funding these two projects, but the historical

patterns have resulted in similar outcomes.

While Louisville Metro deserves a great deal of credit and recognition for championing the release of the historic redlining maps, they have largely failed to address the structural issues around poverty, housing, and crime in their recent budget. This is a perfect example of motion without movement. The city allocated $18 million in new spending for the police department in the 2018 fiscal year budget, but less than $2 million for the rehabilitation of vacant properties through the Affordable Housing Trust Fund.

Disproportionately funding the police department while failing to adequately address vacant properties demonstrates the city's lack of commitment to tackling the legacy of redlining at the structural level, in spite of their progressive rhetoric.

City planners, developers, and nonprofit 501c3 organizations working in Louisville need to view their current projects through a restorative justice framework so that any new planning is carried out within the lens of social justice. A recent article in the Stanford Social Innovation Review encourages anyone working in low-income communities to ask themselves these questions: "Are you aware of and do you value the existing leadership in the community you plan to serve?" and "Do you understand the historical factors that underlie the issues you aim to tackle?"[176]

Now that the redlining documents have been released, Louisville Metro and city planners have an obligation to conduct all new planning within this historic context.

Along with dismantling the racist systems of city planning, zoning, and private lending practices, grass roots activists in Louisville should call for an immediate moratorium on all residential building permits outside I-265 until vacant properties in west Louisville are reduced by one-third. There are over 5,000 vacant properties in Louisville with over 3,000 in the west end.[177] Activists need to demand that the city's budget accommodates for the development of a three-year plan to rehab 1,000 vacant west end properties before spending $1.8 million on a new police headquarters. This act would be an appropriate and proportionate response to acknowledging the legacy of redlining in Louisville.

There are opportunities to create an impact investment fund that is funded by local, state, federal government, foundations, and financial institutions that profited from redlining to invest in formerly redlined areas. These funds could be combined with smaller funding amounts from local residents that allow current residents to profits from the economic redevelopment of their own communities, and ensures a level of equitable development and prevents gentrification.

Activists groups should explore class-action lawsuits against the real estate agencies that created the 1938 maps and the banks that implemented their recommendations. Moreover, activists should encourage the Department of Housing and Urban Development (HUD), the Department of Transportation (DOT), and other federal agencies to reject Louisville Metro applications for water, sewer, and highway projects until the legacies of redlining are addressed.

The redlining maps should be used to initiate a process of truth and reconciliation through long-term economic and policy reparations for those harmed by their impact and justice for the entities that profited from them.

FAIR HOUSING IS ACCESS TO OPPORTUNITY

Kevin Dunlap, Executive Director
REBOUND, Inc.

Carolyn Miller-Cooper, Former Executive Director
Louisville Metro Human Relations Commission

Affirmatively Furthering Fair Housing ("AFFH") is not about "polic[ing] our right to live in the neighborhoods of our choice";. It is about extending that right to all of our citizens by dismantling the lasting effects of decades of systematic race-based segregation in this country.

In her selectively edited excerpt from the Final Rule of AFFH, Bridget Bush truncates what AFFH intends to do: "Specifically, affirmatively furthering fair housing means taking meaningful actions that, taken together, address significant disparities in housing needs and in access to opportunity, replacing segregated living patterns with truly integrated and balanced living patterns, *transforming racially and ethnically concentrated areas of poverty into areas of opportunity, and fostering and maintaining compliance with civil rights and fair housing laws*" (her deletions are italicized).[178]

For far too long and too often, the only "exercise of free choice" in living situation was made by landlords, leasing agents, and loan providers instead of those seeking housing. Segregation in the United States did not simply emerge from the ether. For decades of this country's history, segregation was socially acceptable, legally enforceable, and widely practiced in city planning and residential leasing.

Until made illegal under the Fair Housing Act of 1968, the Federal Housing Authority explicitly practiced a policy of "redlining" when determining which neighborhoods to approve mortgages in, denying and limiting financial services to certain neighborhoods based on solely racial or ethnic composition. Ms. Bush's charge that AFFH is "social engineering" ignores the fact that impoverished communities are already the result of conscious efforts by both local public and private actors to separate particular racial and ethnic groups from the majority population.

Ms. Bush plays upon an ambiguity in the term "steering," attempting to conflate its legal reference to past systematic segregation of communities with contemporary attempts to proactively remedy the damage done by those practices. Doing so ignores the fact that our present reality is (quite literally) built directly upon these past discriminatory actions. Ms. Bush is correct in pointing out that housing discrimination has been illegal since the 1960s; however, the effects of illegal housing discrimination are still acutely felt, precisely because of how rampant and lasting such discriminatory practices were in the past.

Ms. Bush cites New York's Chinatown, Boston's Little Italy, and Chicago's Greek Town as "wonderful ethnic neighborhoods" that would be victimized by the "federally mandated utopia" of AFFH.

However, she neglects to mention that these communities came into being in part due to the very discriminatory practices that the U.S. Department of Housing and Urban Development (HUD) policies attempt to correct with rules such as AFFH (in addition to discrimination based on race, the Fair Housing Act protects against discrimination on the basis of national origin, amongst other categories, such as ethnicity, age, sex, and disability). In fact, this example demonstrates how prior generations' discriminatory practices remain etched into the character and contours of today's neighborhoods.

Choice is necessary but ultimately insufficient on its own to escape poverty. Rather, such behaviors are enabled by communities wherein the grinding effects of endemic poverty do not restrict those options. One's circumstances ought to enable the best choices that one can make, and that is the goal of AFFH.

The only utopia envisioned by AFFH is "overcom[ing] historic patterns of segregation, promote fair housing choice, and foster inclusive communities that are free from discrimination."[179] Segregation negated the ability to choose a better life, and failing to take account of its continuing effects in our community will keep poverty in place. By acknowledging and attempting to remedy the past, AFFH enables these choices, so that the American Dream remains a future for as many people as possible.

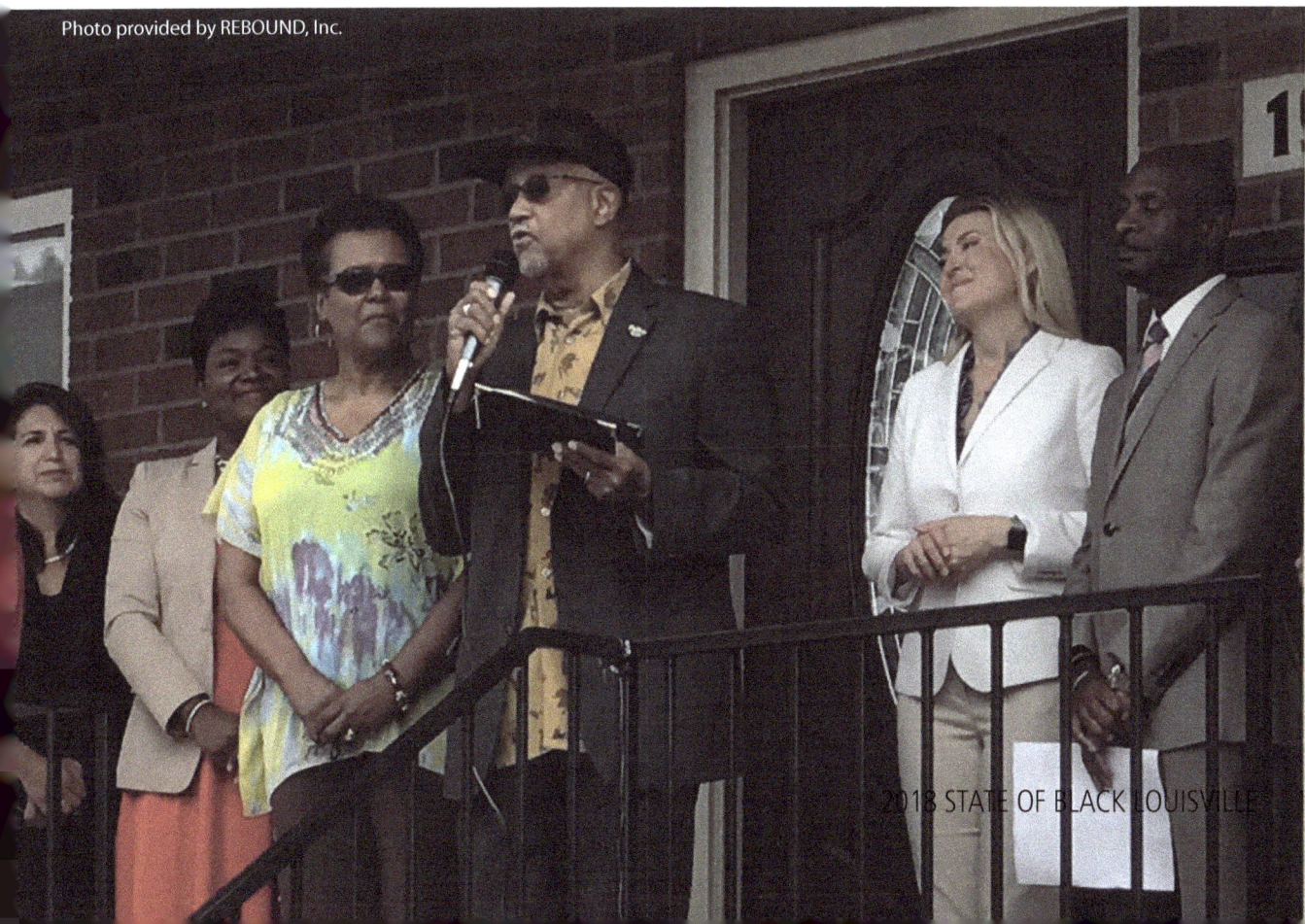

Photo provided by REBOUND, Inc.

A SYSTEMIC BARRIER TO IMPROVING LOW HOMEOWNERSHIP RATES FOR BLACK HOUSEHOLDS IN LOUISVILLE

Cathy Hinko, Executive Director
Metropolitan Housing Coalition

In Louisville, 70% of White households are homeowners, while, in Louisville, 37% of Black/African American households are homeowners.[180] This shocking imbalance encompasses the ability to amass an asset and permanently change economic status as much as it leaves families open to the vicissitudes of the rental market.

Redlining maps, which show the intense racial housing segregation of Louisville, were drawn in the 1930's to instruct mortgage lenders and the real estate industry to treat areas with any concentrations of African Americans as toxic and to avoid investment there. As a result, Blacks were quarantined from the rest of Louisville, including when buying a home. A series of policies on housing lending, including the federal government, denied opportunity for Black households to buy homes in all areas of the city.[181]

The result of these policies is quite evident in the disparity of current homeownership rates. In a report commissioned by the Louisville Human Relations Commission, "Searching for Safe, Fair, and Affordable Housing, Learning from Experiences: An Analysis of Housing Challenges in Louisville Metro," a noticeable set of data emerged in the context of housing. Here you see two charts, one that shows the total population of Louisville by age and sex and one that shows the Black/African American population by age and sex.

The loss of the male Black/African American population between the ages of 25 and 43 goes to the very ability of Black/African American households to change economic class; this affects whole families.

This essay will not delve into the causes that remove Black men of prime earning years from Louisville in such large percentages. While a cursory review of the data on criminal law enforcement shows it is one driving force [182] [183] whatever the cause, the result has severe impacts on housing opportunities for

CHART 1

Age and Sex: Total Population
Louisville/Jefferson County, KY, 2009-2013

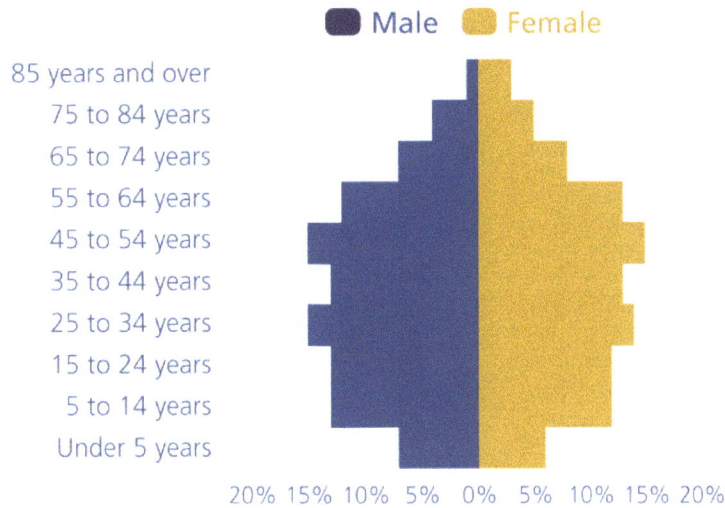

■ Male ■ Female

85 years and over	
75 to 84 years	
65 to 74 years	
55 to 64 years	
45 to 54 years	
35 to 44 years	
25 to 34 years	
15 to 24 years	
5 to 14 years	
Under 5 years	

20% 15% 10% 5% 0% 5% 10% 15% 20%

SOURCE: *U.S. Census, 2009-2013 5-year American Community Survey*

families.[184] With the loss of an adult family member, the impact on the ability of Black/African American families to gain wealth through, for instance, homeownership as well as savings is intuitive.

The data support this intuition. In Louisville, the median income for male, full-time workers were 20% higher than their female counterparts. A family with one wage earner, particularly a female wage earner, has a higher rate of poverty. In Louisville, 24% of families with children live in poverty, but 67% of those families in poverty are single, female-headed households.

We know that married couples have a homeownership rate of 83% in Louisville compared to female-headed households with an ownership rate 42%. Clearly, removing men from their families during prime child-rearing years has a direct effect on the ability of the family to own.

With the loss specifically of Black men – this significant loss of a percentage of the population is

not true for Whites – Black families will, perforce, have a higher rate of poverty. In Louisville, poverty for Blacks is 31% compared to 12% for White residents.

Without full income, a family becomes limited in where they can live in Louisville. For those families lucky enough to get a Section 8 Voucher (as of October 2017, there are over 18,000 households on the waiting list), the notion of being able to live anywhere is illusory. The Voucher Payment Standard only makes the bottom 40% of units financially available with subsidy. Most of those units are in a very small geographic area (see attached maps). Without a voucher there is absolutely no ability to move to most geographic areas of Louisville.

POLICY IMPLICATIONS

There are many policy recommendations concerning fair criminal justice practices, from policing to the administration of the courts, and these are clearly important in this context as well. I will defer to those experts. There are also policy recommendations to achieve equal pay for equal work, addressing

CHART 2

Age and Sex: Black/African-American Population

Louisville/Jefferson County, KY, 2009-2013

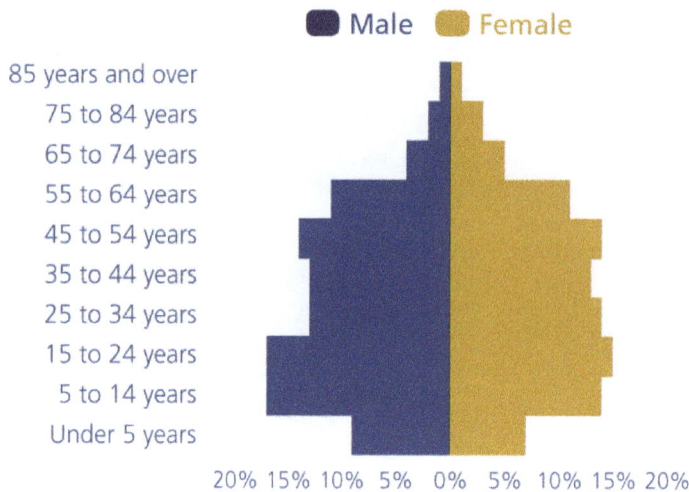

■ Male ● Female

85 years and over
75 to 84 years
65 to 74 years
55 to 64 years
45 to 54 years
35 to 44 years
25 to 34 years
15 to 24 years
5 to 14 years
Under 5 years

20% 15% 10% 5% 0% 5% 10% 15% 20%

SOURCE: *U.S. Census, 2009-2013 5-year American Community Survey*

both sex and gender differences and those also are important in this context and, again, I defer to those experts.

Having united families with sufficient income is the best way to address our problems of segregation and wealth disparities, but there are some short-term policies affecting housing that should be adopted as we work for equality in pay and treatment in criminal justice.

First, change the Section 8 Voucher Program to ensure that Payment Standards, which dictate the amount of money a family can spend on both housing and utilities without being cost-burdened, factors in fair housing goals as well as affordable housing goals. If not, we will continue to see the concentrations of people in protected classes in small geographic areas, even when the family is being assisted. Since Voucher payments can also be used to help pay a mortgage, the amount of the Payment Standard has even more reach than making different geographic areas available to assisted families.

Next, for those unassisted, homeownership programs that are designed for single-income households need to be developed. Currently, single adults with children must conform to lending practices based on outdated models of married family and income structure; household composition has been shown to have changed.

Lastly, use Louisville Affordable Housing Trust Fund dollars to achieve fair housing standards. Create ownership opportunities within financial reach in areas that are concentrated by race, poverty and female-headed households. Create rental opportunities that are affordable in areas that are all White, higher income and ownership, as well as ownership opportunities that use smaller lot sizes.

All resources of Louisville Metro government used in housing and neighborhood development should also address fair housing goals to alieve concentrations of affordable housing in small areas and ensure meaningful affordable housing opportunities in all areas of Louisville.

BLACK LOUISVILLE'S HOUSING CRISIS

Chanelle Helm, Lead Core Organizer
"SCZ", Core Organizer
Black Lives Matter Louisville

Black Lives Matter (BLM) Louisville is a collective of Black and Brown organizers who work in a fusion for Black Louisville to build and raise up our communities from our different platforms. While maintaining our various scopes, we can affirm that #AllBlackLivesMatter.

From the Ferguson uprising, the Visions of Abolition after Trayvon Martin's death, and the shoulders of many Black activists in this city, we have maintained the work of Black liberation. With the goal of avenging our ancestors, we also fight for: reparations; abolition of the police; "Free the Land", which is saturated with our blood, sweat, and tears; justice against food apartheids; and rights to education and housing.

Over the past four years, our organizing has revealed several issues in and around Black Louisville – most issues too old to repair. We understand that reform is a promise, but it is not one we can rely on to sustain Black people, Black bodies, or to produce Black liberation. We believe in building new systems built on principles that support the transformation of Black lives.

We have four main teams that support the work of Black Louisville communities: education, healing, housing, and police accountability. Each team is a collective of organizers within BLM Louisville and our social justice coalition Stand Up Sunday, along with Black Louisville community leaders and support leaders who help build work around our manifestos and goals. Each team has led extensive work. These include: pushing policy change at Jefferson County Public Schools (JCPS); fighting against the good old boy system within the Louisville Metro Police Department (LMPD); creating the Mae Street healing clinic; supporting renters in their time of need; providing bail to those targeted by the judicial system; and forcing the Lincoln Village Regional Juvenile Detention Center to close after the death of Gynnya McMillen.

While our teams grow and tactics strengthen (our healing team and Freedom Academy are currently being funded), we stay committed to the #staylowandbuild, understanding the foundation that eliminates the root causes of our oppression. From our network, Black Lives Matter is an ideological and political intervention in a world where Black lives are systematically and intentionally targeted for demise. It is an affirmation of Black folks' contributions to this society, our humanity, and our resilience in the face of deadly oppression.

That deadly serum in the underbelly of oppression is the housing crisis of Black Louisville. Evictions are increasing in area, according to a report by the Metropolitan Housing Coalition.[185] There is predatory selling of rental homes that are displacing young families. Disabled community members are at risk of eviction every other week. Abandoned homes are being taken over by outside developers. The housing crisis in Black Louisville is one that could be solved by financial literacy, but #staylowandbuild is to house people.

Our housing team began in December of 2016. The mission is to combat generational poverty and marginalization of homeownership that exists for Black people in the city. Historical and structural racism are barriers to individual and community ownership of resources that allow us to practice greater self-determination. We believe a foundation for racial justice and equity begins when wealth is redistributed and reparations are given by people who have historically benefited from systems of White supremacy, colonialism, and capitalism.

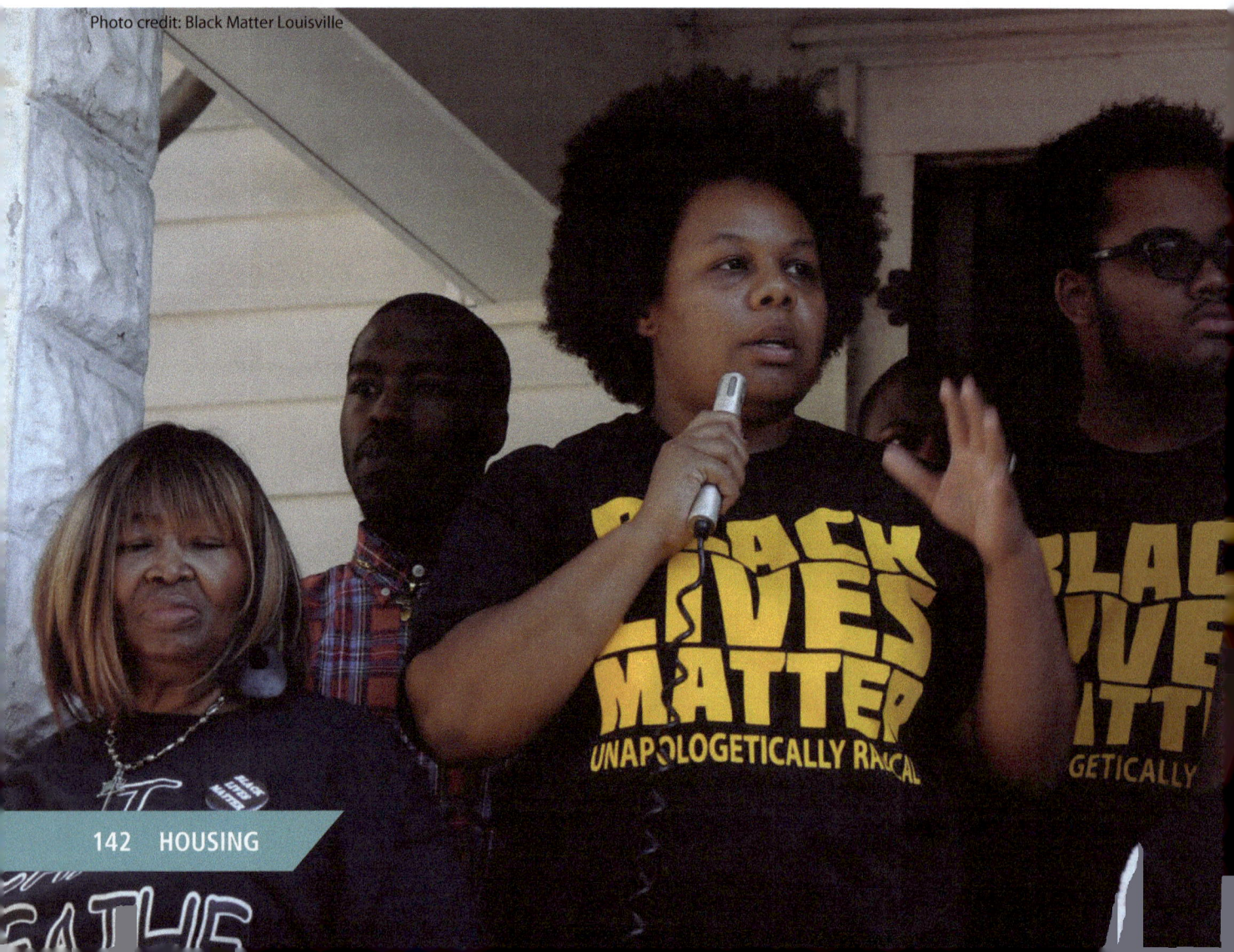

Photo credit: Black Matter Louisville

Our housing team works to find properties that could be purchased with the goal of individual family ownership, or spaces that could be developed for the use of community infrastructure. We focus on properties with abandonment, pre-abandonment, and tax liens, so we reduce the number of vacant properties in our community while keeping the needed resources to invest relatively low.

This increases the possibilities for Black families to acquire property from us at no or little cost as well as the boundless possibilities for impacted community members who seek communal ventures to minimize their start-up capital on property. Our funding is supplied by White donors who know that reparations are real and that property obtainment has been a continual White supremacist tactic to eliminate Black people from the very communities we have built.

Black Louisville has created a historical infrastructure in Louisville. It has been denounced, ignored, and thrown away in a possible city that intends to grow from an anti-Black foundation. We declare that Black Louisville cannot undergo mass displacement. We will stand with our community members and fight for just housing with a desire to find a home. We stand on the shoulders of our ancestors to acquire and free the land.

FORGE ADVANTAGES FOR MILLENNIAL HOMEBUYERS WHILE REDEVELOPING GREAT NEIGHBORHOODS

Kevin Dunlap, Executive Director
REBOUND, Inc.
Lisa Thompson, Chief Impact Officer
Louisville Urban League

Let's look forward.

Louisville is challenged to compete for the investment attention of African American millennials – those born in Louisville and tempted to leave, and others who could choose Louisville as a 21st century place to invest their time and talent.

Louisville Urban League and its affiliate, REBOUND, Inc, are experienced community-based developers leaning forward into this dramatic generational shift positioning to offer millennial homebuyers an array of amazing choices.

Millennials were born between the early 1980s to the early 2000s. If this isn't you, then it's the texting creature who handles your investment portfolio or is prepping you for surgery while cruising Instagram. Millennials are urbane, politically savvy, and educated. They are far more diverse and outnumber baby boomers. Between 14 and 25 percent of America's millennials are African American who are leading users of electronic media. They are technologic trailblazers across the last decade's digital divide. Delayed in home purchases by student and consumer debt, this generation is eager to begin the next stage of their lives.

Their children will outnumber them and will be the epitome of the American Dream – the first majority-minority generation in the nation's history.

LOUISVILLE COMPETES FOR MILLENNIAL CHOICE

Does Louisville want to compete for their home-buying investments? REBOUND, Inc., certainly does, and if we work together as a community, there is an innovative way we can redevelop the past while capturing disproportionate market share of this forward-looking generation – and their beautiful children.

For the first time in nearly a century, Louisville's nine western neighborhoods are transforming themselves, preparing for new life and opportunities. Over $800 million in new financial capital is in the development pipeline headed to west Louisville. Revitalization is in full swing in neighborhoods east of downtown with Smoketown, Shelby Park, and Germantown gaining market traction. New price points in these neighborhoods now limit access to some potential buyers.

Media is already covering exciting work in neighborhoods that border downtown to the west. We want to ensure people who already make these neighborhoods great are afforded opportunities to share in transformations and wealth development. Future positive change must include Louisville's African American millennials. And, we need to create national campaigns that invite relocating millennials to choose Louisville.

Healthy markets are made up of neighborhoods where it makes sense to confidently invest time and talent with a fair expectation of a return on investment. Now, more than ever, it's time to rally every bold effort to accelerate revitalization by making it possible for legacy families to remain and for entry-level professionals to own a piece of what will be a rapidly changing housing market.

Who has been priced out of other markets? Teachers, medical technicians and health care workers, peace keepers, and returning military veterans want both a home and a community. If we invite them, they may want to call Louisville home, and the western neighborhoods their community.

As millennials round the first life turn and enter the home-buying stretch, they have a few dwelling demands. Let's be wise and listen so that this influential group can choose Louisville's diverse and rebounding neighborhoods. Many are saddled with debt like no other generation before them due to the high costs of their education, so cost-conscious quality is key. They are likely to buy as single people who are mindful that their household

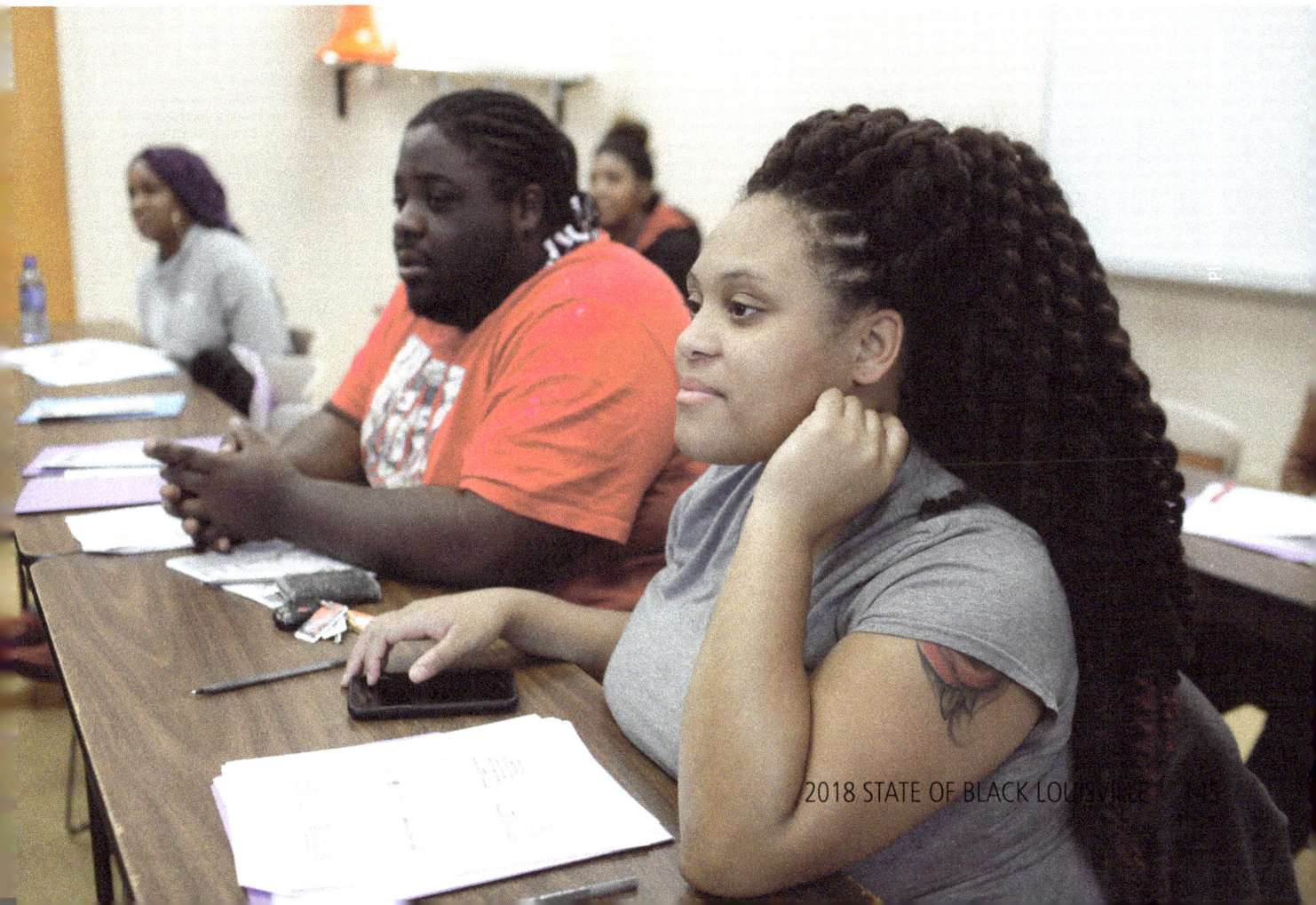

will expand before they sell, so design that allows for life change is more than an amenity (think shotgun and bungalow renovations with additions of great room space and parking pads). They like the thought of flipping for profit, but most are better at fixing a computer than a faucet, so they look for turn-key housing with enhancement opportunity. The quick access to highways and traffic corridors of Portland, Russell, and Shawnee neighborhoods are not lost on these intrepid investors.

REBOUND and the Louisville Urban League are listening and ready to partner with others who care about 21st century home quality. Both organizations have long histories of working with grassroots and resident groups to make big visions come to life.

REBOUND IS A NEIGHBORHOOD MARKET-BUILDER

Launched by the Louisville Urban League, REBOUND, Inc. began as a not-for-profit public/private partnership to develop new single-family homes in the Russell neighborhood and to attract other housing developers into the neighborhood by proving that a homeownership market did exist. This initiative was seeded with generous support and technical advice from Humana Founder David Jones, Sr. In its first strategy, 47 homes were built and sold by REBOUND and five new housing developers came to the neighborhood.

REBOUND is now a federally designated Community Housing Development Organization (CHDO). This allows REBOUND to work with philanthropy as well as leverage far more housing impact with public funding and private financing. REBOUND's second strategy launched in 2010 acquired, rehabbed, and sold another 41 single family homes in the Russell, Shawnee, Chickasaw, Newburg, Hallmark and Shively neighborhoods. This not only produced quality homes in great neighborhoods for fine families; it established comparable market values to lift appraisal results.

THE 21ST CENTURY LOUISVILLE URBAN LEAGUE

The Louisville Urban League is a not-for-profit, nonpartisan, interracial community development and service organization dedicated to eliminating racism and its adverse impacts on the regional community. Our mission is to help African Americans and other marginalized people to attain social and economic equality through a five-point strategy of jobs, justice, education, health and housing. The Louisville Urban League was a revitalization innovator when it successfully developed a $2.2 million commercial building on West Broadway. This investment was bold, staking the agency's future on a venture that was both ahead of its time and successful. Soon, new investment of over $70 million will arrive on West Broadway as Passport and YMCA relocate.

Earlier this year, the U.S. Department of Housing and Urban Development chose the Russell neighborhood for a Choice Neighborhood Initiative Grant, which can leverage $200 million to transform the Beecher Terrace apartment community. The League continues to drive the change momentum as the developer of the Heritage West site where a $30 million state-of-the-art facility which will restore Louisville's national prestige as a track and field destination.

LOOK FORWARD AND TAKE ACTION

REBOUND is gearing up for a third strategic wave and needs partners, including neighborhood leaders, who want to ensue Louisville is enriched with the talents and compassion of America's millennial generation. New housing impact projects are moving to construction phase soon, designed with millennial lifestyles in mind. REBOUND and Louisville Urban League see a 21st century that values and rehabilitates the best of the past but does not carry forward divisions that can't be allowed to undermine future prosperity that could and should be shared.

Have a millennial in your life? Tell them "Choose Louisville!"

ADDITIONAL CONTRIBUTORS

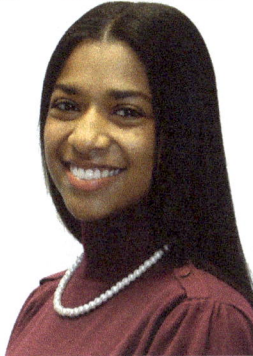

ASHLI FINDLEY, Editor

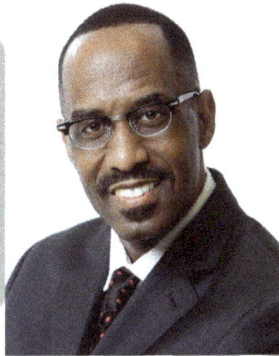

DR. KEVIN COSBY, St. Stephen Church

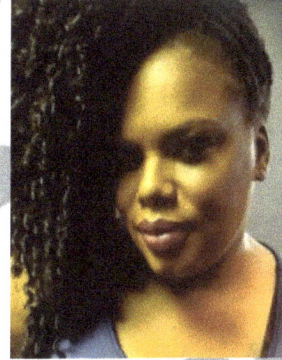

HANNAH DRAKE, Poet

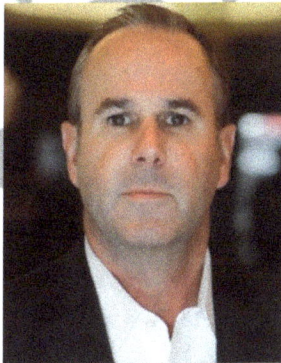

MARC MURPHY, Cartoonist

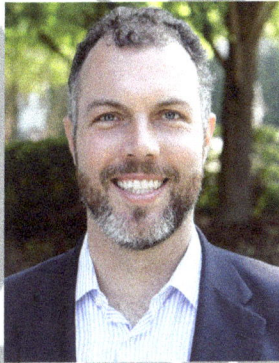

BEN RENO-WEBER, Greater Louisville Project

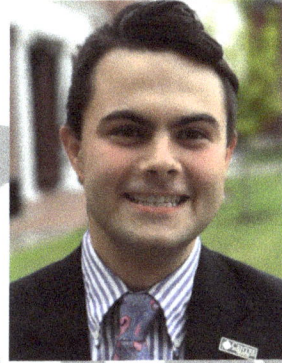

HARRISON KIRBY, Greater Louisville Project

ADDITIONAL DATA

Several contributors provided additional data to better contextualize the information provided throughout this book. That data is compiled her for further reference.

Measure Two: HOUSING SEGREGATION

Map 15: Percentage of Population Identifying as Black or African-American
by Census Tracts – Louisville/Jefferson County 2010–2014

- 0% – 5%
- 6% – 10%
- 11% – 25%
- 26% – 50%
- 51% – 99%
- R/ECAP* Tracts

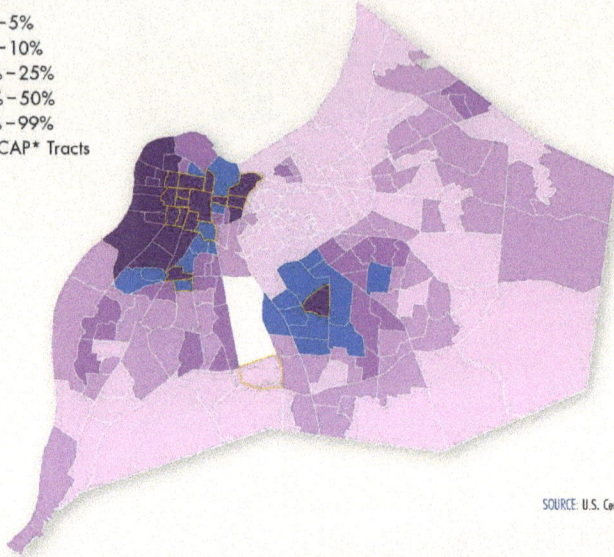

SOURCE: U.S. Census, 2010-2014 5-year American Community Survey
*HUD 2016d. "R/ECAP Tract Current and Historic."

Living In Community | Metropolitan Housing Coalition
metropolitanhousing.org | 2016 State of Metropolitan Housing Report

Measure Two: HOUSING SEGREGATION

Map 14: Percentage of Total Population in Poverty
by Census Tracts – Louisville/Jefferson County 2010–2014

- 0% – 5%
- 6% – 10%
- 11% – 25%
- 26% – 50%
- 51% – 86%
- R/ECAP* Tracts

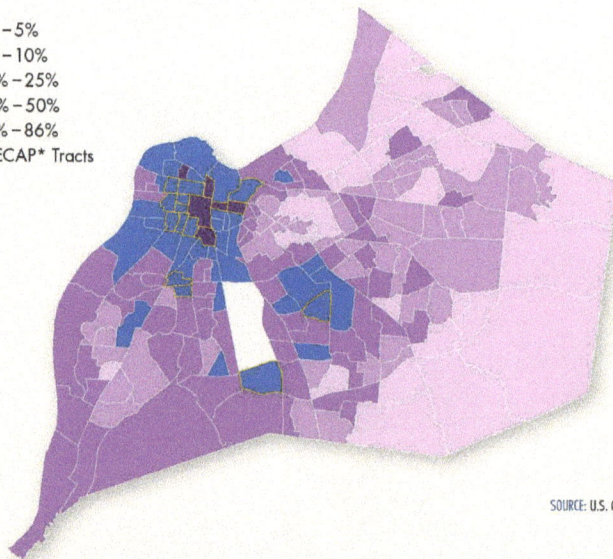

SOURCE: U.S. Census, 2010-2014 5-year American Community Survey
*HUD 2016d. "R/ECAP Tract Current and Historic."

Living In Community | Metropolitan Housing Coalition
metropolitanhousing.org | 2016 State of Metropolitan Housing Report

Figure 4: Percentage of Total Public Housing and Section 8 Units
by Louisville Metro Council Districts – 2016

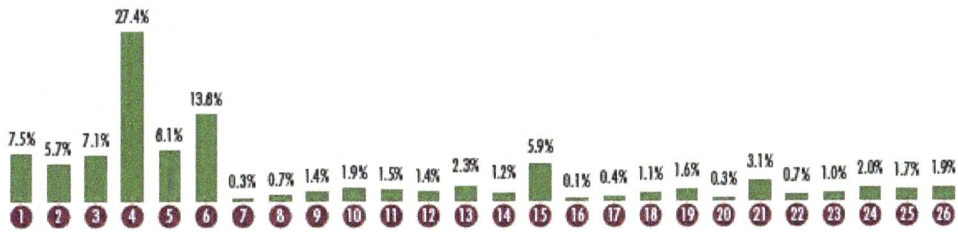

7.5% 1 5.7% 2 7.1% 3 27.4% 4 6.1% 5 13.6% 6 0.3% 7 0.7% 8 1.4% 9 1.9% 10 1.5% 11 1.4% 12 2.3% 13 1.2% 14 5.9% 15 0.1% 16 0.4% 17 1.1% 18 1.6% 19 0.3% 20 3.1% 21 0.7% 22 1.0% 23 2.0% 24 1.7% 25 1.9% 26

Map 2: Subsidized Section 8 Housing
by Louisville Metro Council Districts – 2015

- Section 8 Housing Choice Vouchers
- Project-Based Section 8

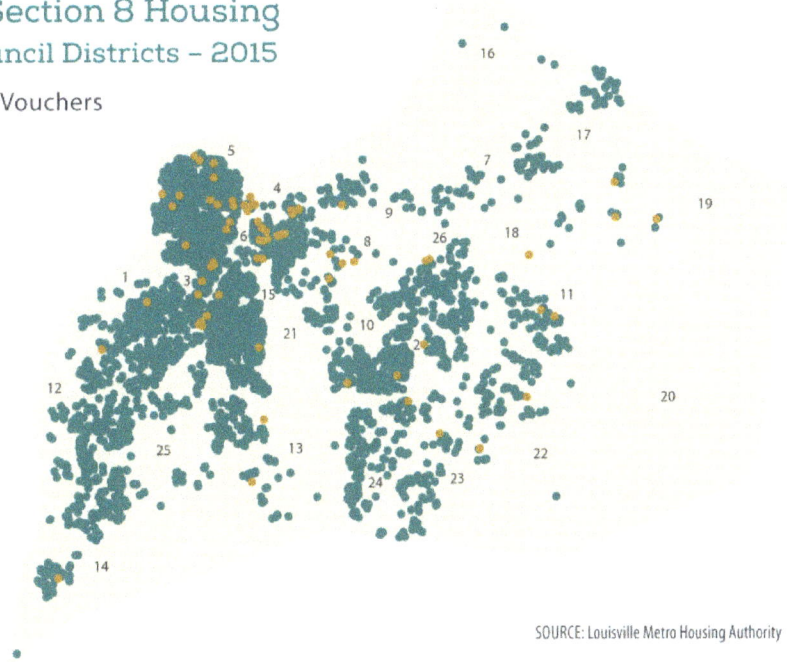

SOURCE: Louisville Metro Housing Authority

Female Unemployment Rate in Louisville

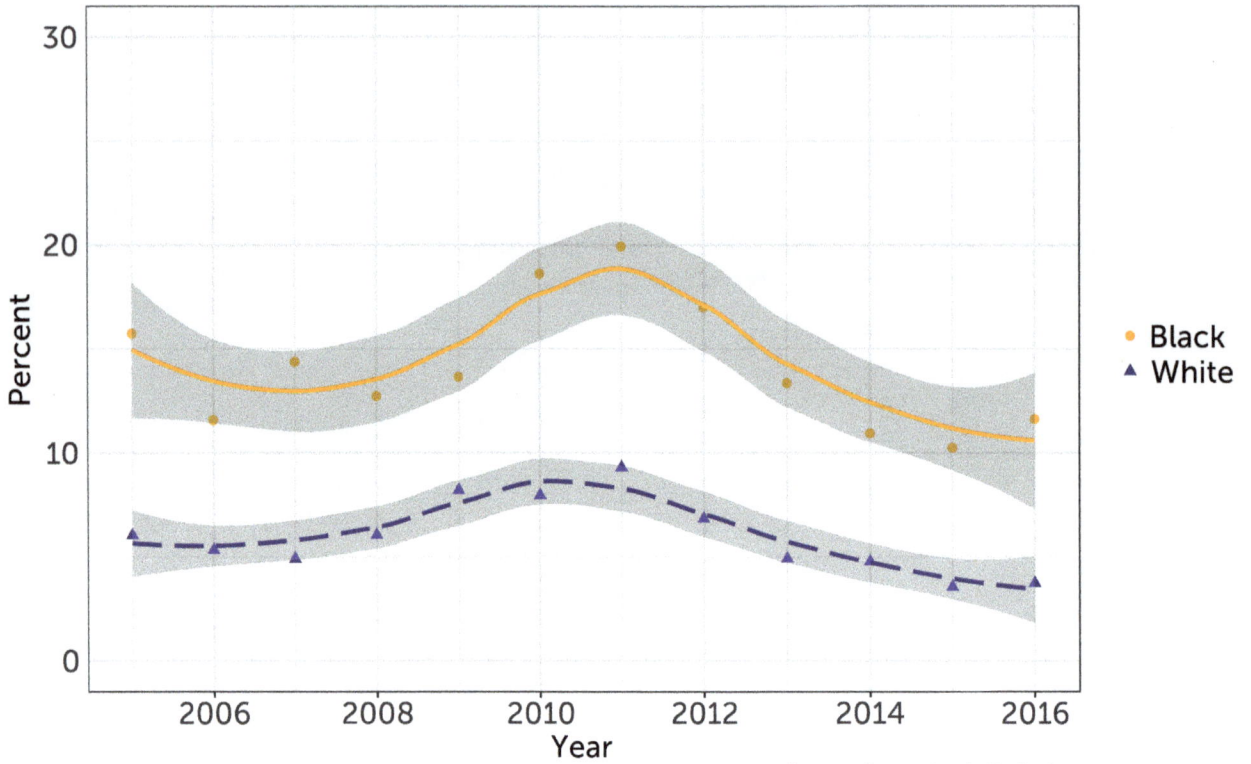

Source: Greater Louisville Project
Data from the American Community Survey, Tables B23002A and B23002B

Median Female Earnings for Full-Time, Year-Round Workers in Louisville

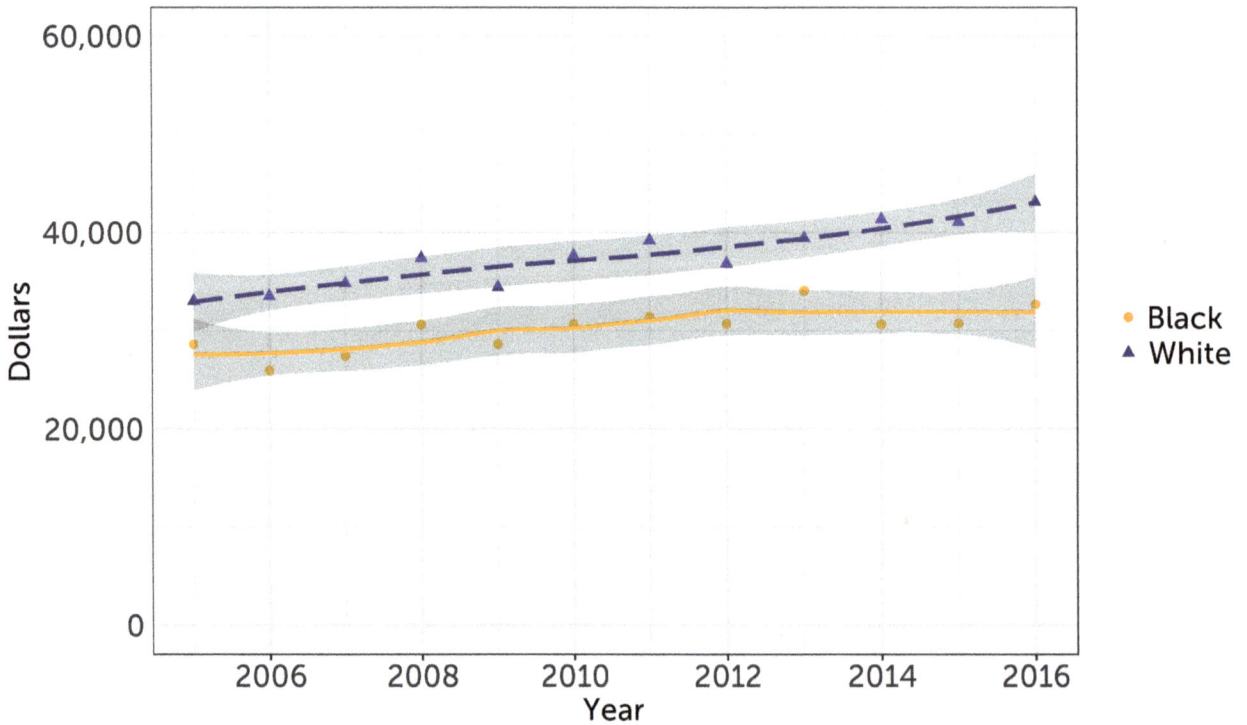

Source: Greater Louisville Project
Data from the American Community Survey, Tables B20017A and B200172B

Median Female Earnings in Louisville

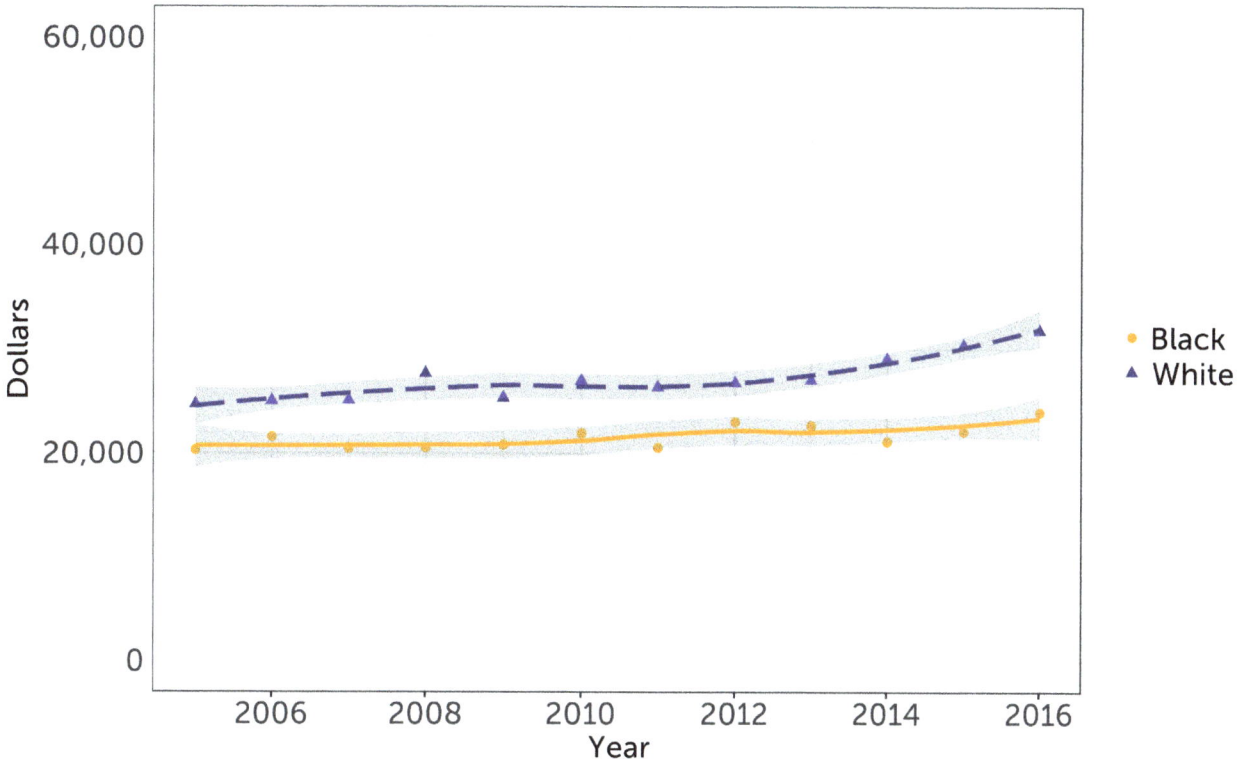

Source: Greater Louisville Project
Data from the American Community Survey, Tables B20017A and B200172B

White Out of Labor Force Rate in Louisville, Ages 24-55

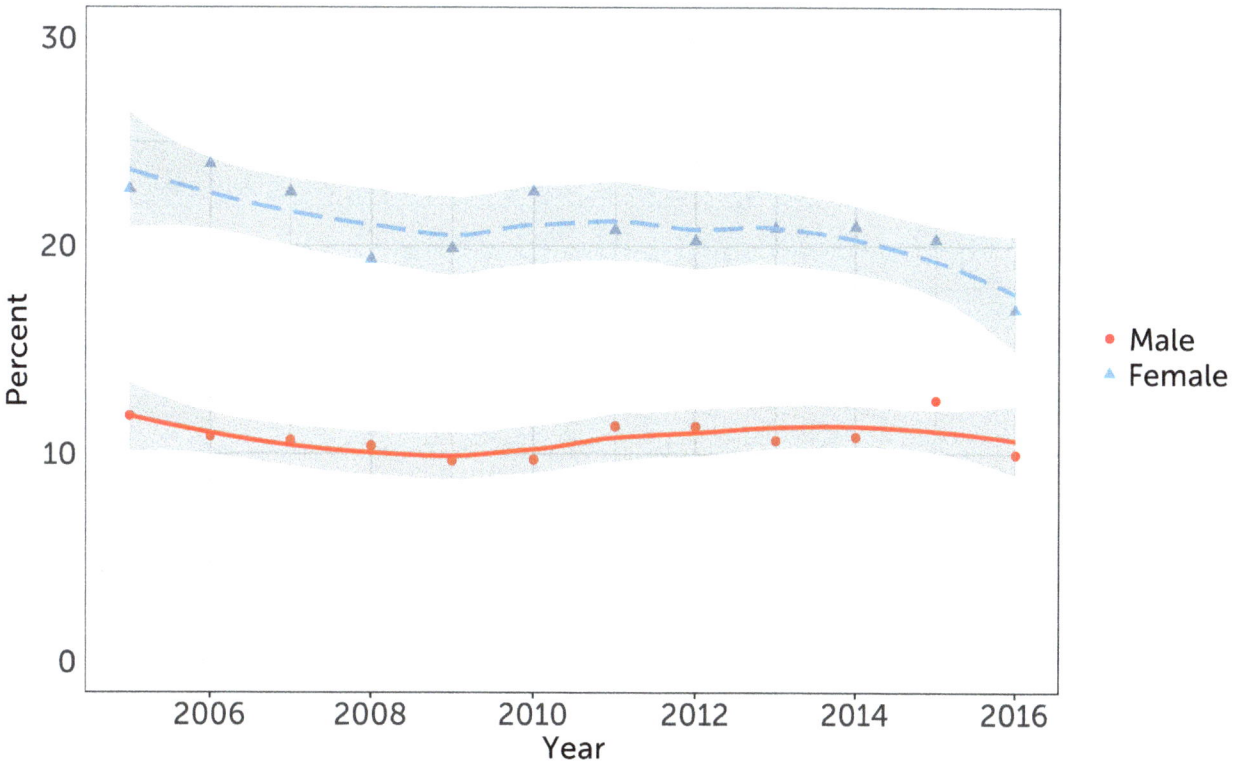

Source: Greater Louisville Project
Data from the American Community Survey, Tables B23002A and B23002B

Male Unemployment Rate in Louisville

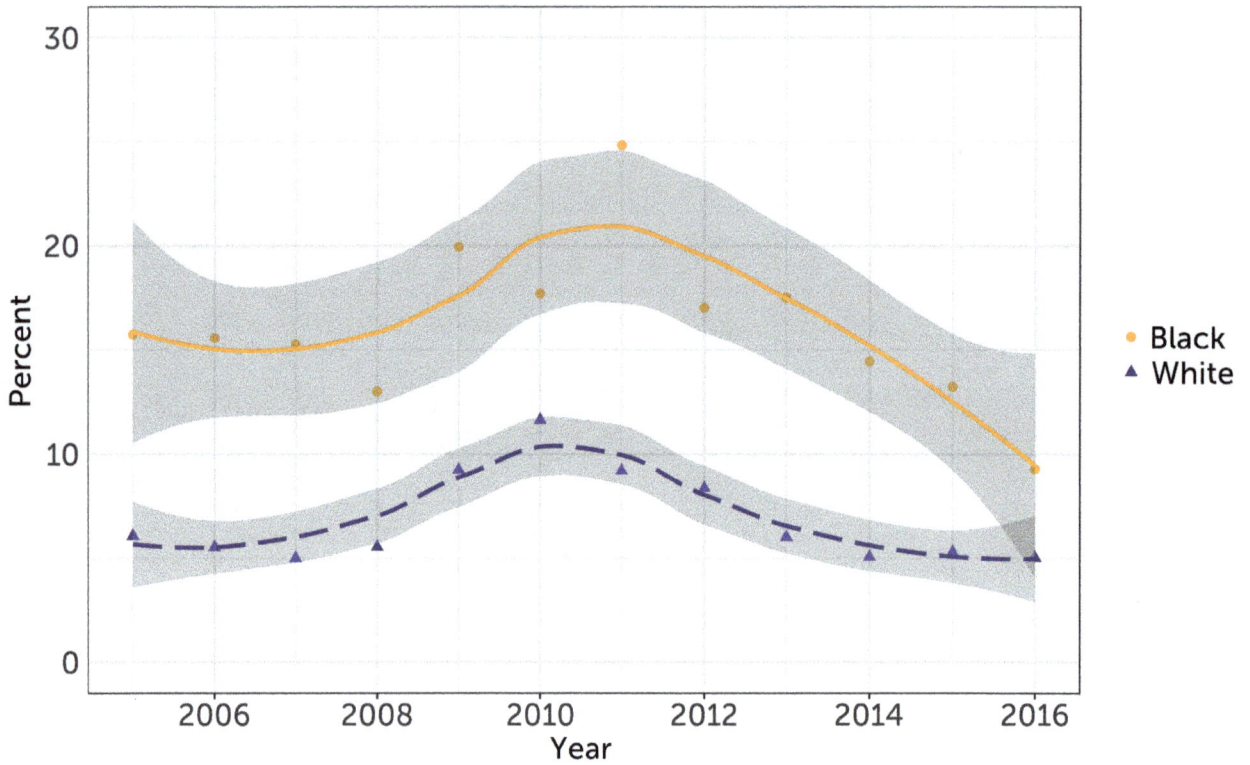

Source: Greater Louisville Project
Data from the American Community Survey, Tables B23002A and B23002B

Median Male Earnings in Louisville

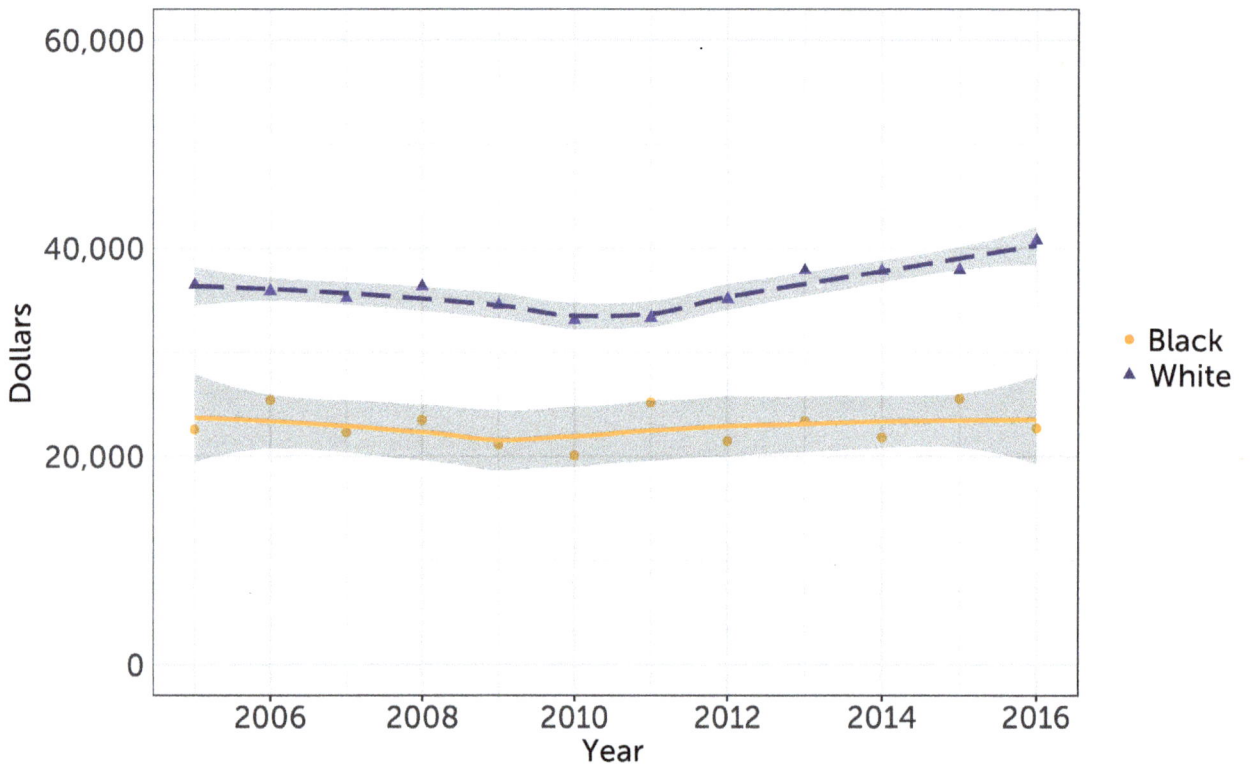

Source: Greater Louisville Project
Data from the American Community Survey, Tables B20017A and B200172B

Median Male Earnings for Full-Time, Year-Round Workers in Louisville

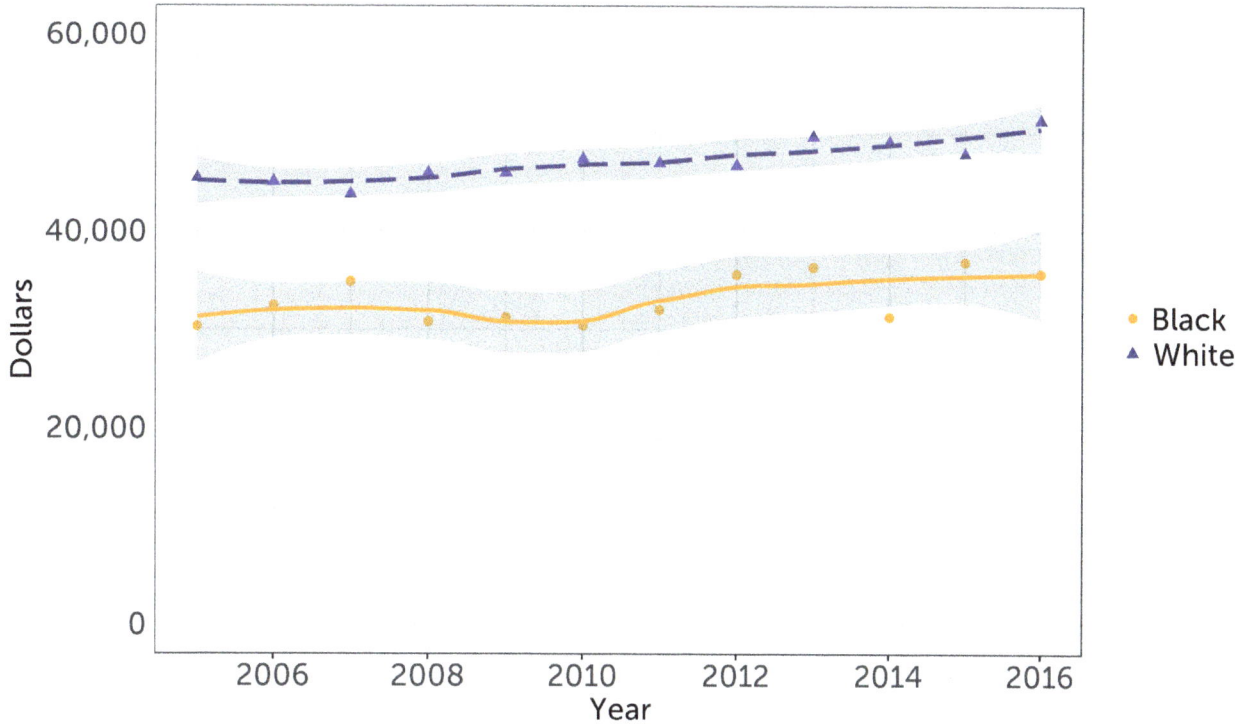

Source: Greater Louisville Project
Data from the American Community Survey, Tables B20017A and B200172B

Black Out of Labor Force Rate in Louisville, Ages 24-55

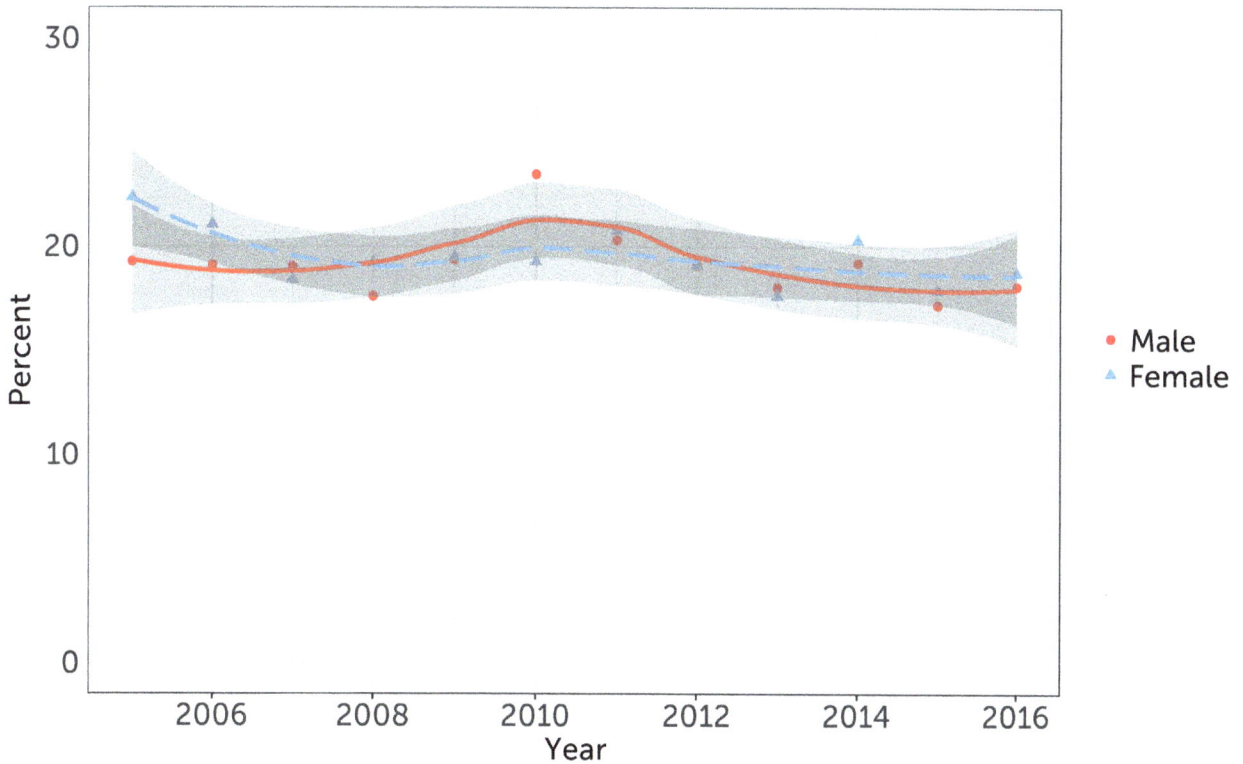

Source: Greater Louisville Project
Data from the American Community Survey, Tables B23002A and B23002B

Poverty Rate in Louisville

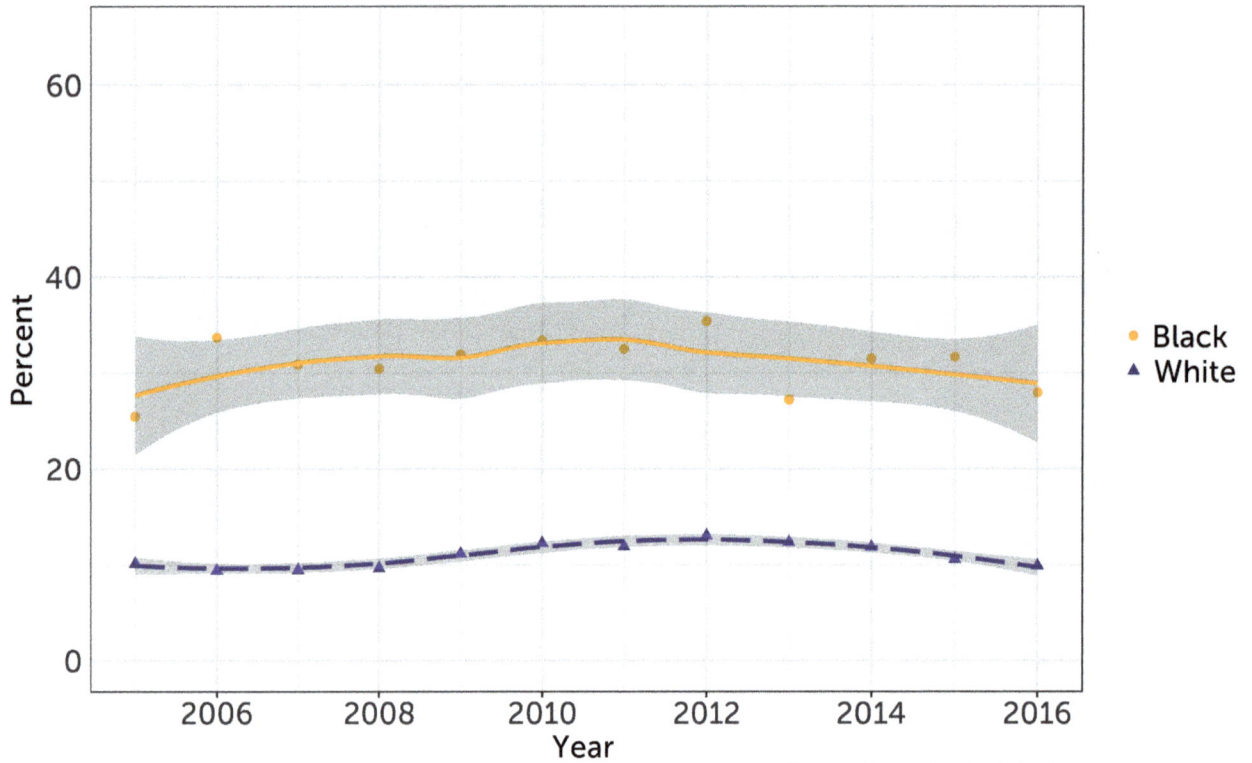

Source: Greater Louisville Project
Data from the American Community Survey, Tables B17001A and B17001B

Child Poverty Rate in Louisville

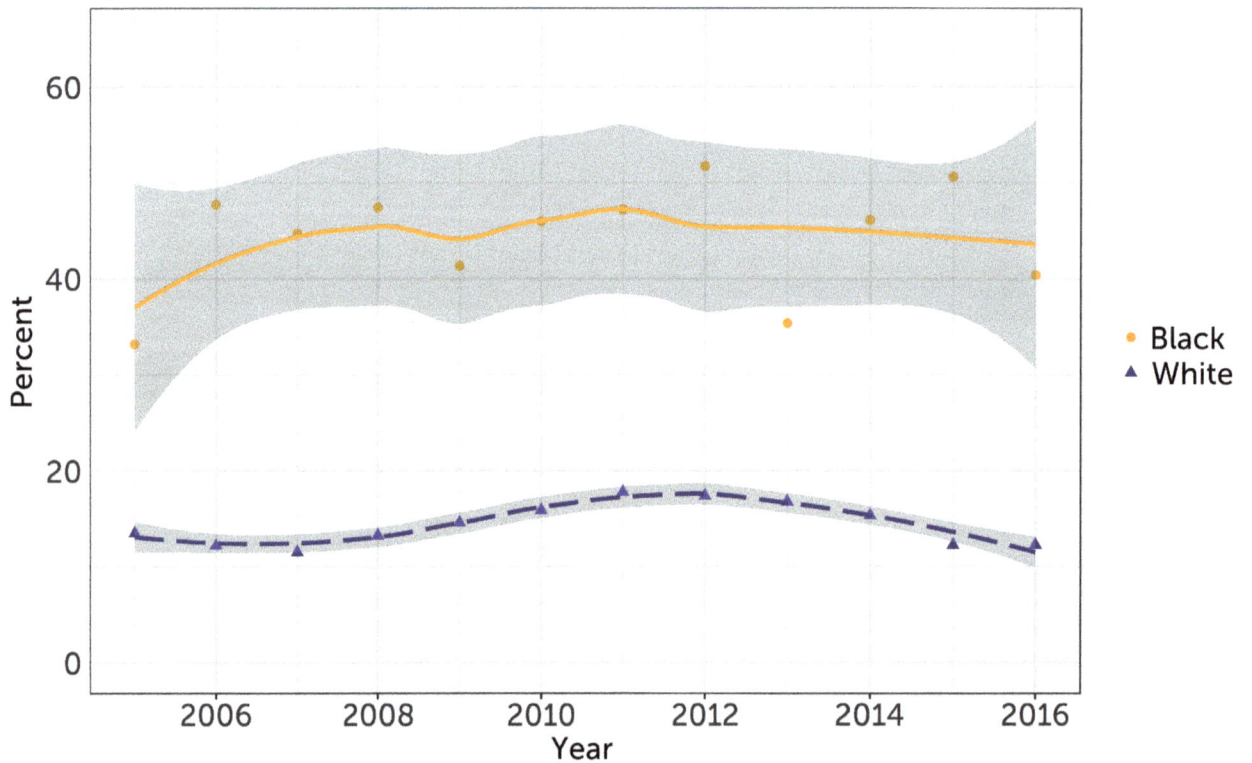

Source: Greater Louisville Project
Data from the American Community Survey, Tables B17001A and B17001B

Highest Level of Educational Attainment in Lousville by Race and Gender, 2011-2016

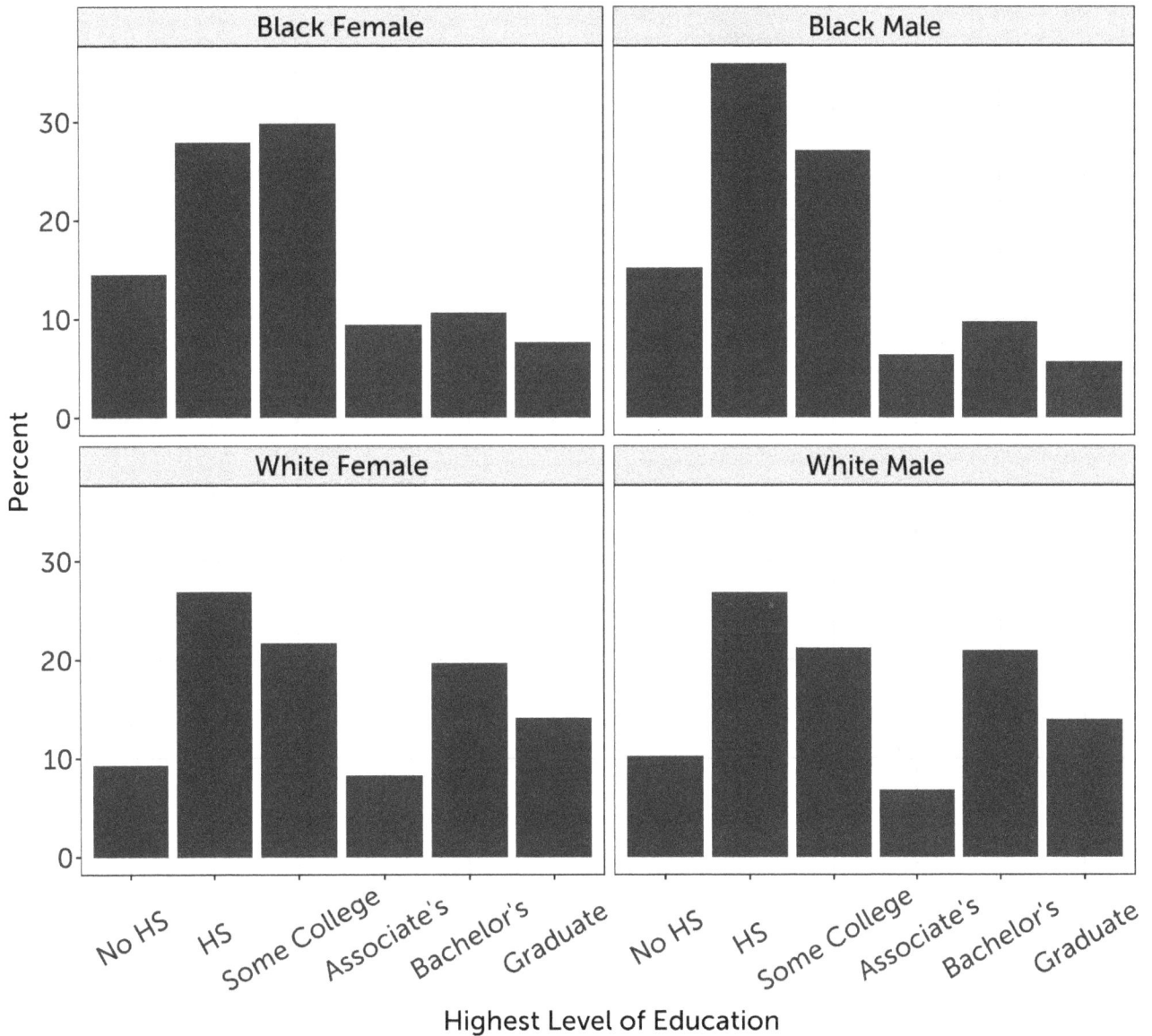

Source: Greater Louisville Project
Data from the American Community Survey, Tables B15002A and B15002B

ENDNOTES

1   Jackson, T.F. (2007). *From civil rights to human rights: Martin Luther King, Jr., and the struggle for economic justice,* 348. Philadelphia, PA: University of Pennsylvania Press.

2   Johnson, L.B. (1965, June 4). *Commencement address at Howard University: 'To fulfill these rights.'* Accessible at http://www.presidency.ucsb.edu/ws/?pid=27021

3   Lipsitz, G. (1998). *The possessive investment in whiteness: How white people profit from identity politics.* Philadelphia, PA: Temple University Press.

4   City-Data. (2013). *Louisville, Kentucky poverty rate data* [Data file]. Retrieved from http://www.city-data.com/poverty/poverty-Louisville-Kentucky.html

5   U.S. Census Bureau. (2016). *2016 American Community Survey.* Retrieved from https://factfinder.census.gov/.

6   Lee, H., McCormick, T., Hicken, M.T., & Wildeman, C. (2016). Measuring the social impact of mass imprisonment on America's black and white families and communities. *Scholars Strategy Network.* Retrieved from http://www.scholarsstrategynetwork.org/brief/measuring-social-impact-mass-imprisonment-americas-black-and-white-families-and-communities

7   Claritas. Healthy Louisville. (2017). *Summary data for county: Jefferson* [Data file]. Retrieved from http://www.healthylouisvillemetro.org/index.php?module=DemographicData&controller=index&action=index

8   Zip Atlas. (2017). *Percentage of blacks (African Americans in Louisville, KY by zip code* [Data file]. Retrieved from http://zipatlas.com/us/ky/louisville/zip-code-comparison/percentage-black-population.htm

9   U.S. Census Bureau. (2017). *Current population demographics and statistics for Kentucky by age, gender and race* [Data file]. Suburban Stats. Retrieved from https://suburbanstats.org/population/how-many-people-live-in-kentucky

10   Glowick, M. (2014, November 18). Study: Black arrest rate higher across region. *The Courier-Journal.* Retrieved from http://www.courier-journal.com/story/news/local/2014/11/18/study-black-arrest-rate-higher-across-region/19249311/

11   Howard, K. (2016). Kentucky 3rd in nation in barring felons from the voting booth. *WFPL News Louisville.* Retrieved from http://wfpl.org/kentucky-3rd-in-nation-in-barring-felons-from-the-voting-booth/

12   Claritas. (2017). *Summary data for county: Jefferson* [Data file]. Retrieved from http://www.healthylouisvillemetro.org/index.php?module=DemographicData&controller=index&action=index

13   University of Louisville Institutional Research and Planning. (2016, June 8). *Incumbency v. estimated availability summary* [Data file]. Louisville, KY: University of Louisville.

14   Zip Atlas. (2017). *Percentage of blacks (African Americans) in Louisville, KY by zip code* [Data file]. Retrived from http://zipatlas.com/us/ky/louisville/zip-code-comparison/percentage-black-population.htm

15   Emmons, W. R. & Noeth, B.J. (2015). The demographics of wealth: How age, education and race separate thrivers from strugglers in today's economy, essay No. 2. *Federal Reserve Bank of St. Louis.* Retrieved from https://www.stlouisfed.org/household-financial-stability/the-demographics-of-wealth/essay-2-the-role-of-education

16   Boshara, R. (2017, April 12). Black college graduates are losing wealth. Here's what can help. *The Washington Post.* Retrieved from https://www.washingtonpost.com/opinions/black-college-graduates-are-losing-wealth-heres-what-can-help/2017/04/12/cd83ba64-1ba4-11e7-9887-1a5314b56a08_story.html?utm_term=.196aad8b3c91

17   U.S. Census Bureau. (2016). *2011-2015 American Community Survey 5 Year Estimate.* Retrieved from https://factfinder.census.gov/.

18   Kentucky Center for Economic Policy. (N.D.). *Our commonwealth: A primer on the Kentucky state budget.* Retrieved from http://kypolicy.org/dash/wp-content/uploads/2016/01/Ky-Budget-Primer-2016-web-ready.pdf

19   Office of State Budget Director. (2013, February 5). *Governor Beshear's blue ribbon commission on tax reform.* Retrieved from https://osbd.ky.gov/Publications/Documents/Presentations/130205_ARPresentation_BlueRibbonTaxCommission.pdf

20   Kentucky Center for Economic Policy. (2014). *The state of working Kentucky*. Retrieved from https://kypolicy.org/dash/wp-content/uploads/2014/08/State-of-Working-KY-2014-final.pdf

21   Kentucky Center for Economic Policy. (2014). *The state of working Kentucky*. Retrieved from https://kypolicy.org/dash/wp-content/uploads/2014/08/State-of-Working-KY-2014-final.pdf

22   Kentuckians For The Commonwealth. (N.D.). *Kentucky Forward Plan: Fair and sensible tax reform*. Retrieved from http://kftc.org/issues/kentucky-forward-plan

23   Blackford, L. (2017, January 3). Kentucky's tax code gives more money than it collects. Would reform change that? *Lexington Herald-Leader*. Retrieved from http://www.kentucky.com/news/local/education/article123741909.html

24   Kentucky Educational Television. (N.D.). *Kentucky tonight: Tax reform*. Retrieved from https://www.ket.org/episode/KKYTO%20002419/

25   Office of State Budget Director. (2018). *2016-2018 Budget of the commonwealth: Budget in brief: Distribution of general fund appropriations*. Retrieved from https://osbd.ky.gov/Publications/Documents/Budget%20Documents/2016-2018%20Executive%20Budget%20Recommendation/Budget%20in%20Brief.pdf

26   Prison Policy Initiative. (2010). *Overrepresentation of blacks in Kentucky*. Retrieved from https://www.prisonpolicy.org/graphs/2010percent/KY_Blacks_2010.html

27   Dakwar, J. & Turner, J. (2014, October 27). Racial disparities in sentencing: Hearing on reports of racism in the justice system of the United States. *American Civil Liberties Union*. Retrieved from https://www.aclu.org/sites/default/files/assets/141027_iachr_racial_disparities_aclu_submission_0.pdf

28   The New York Times Editorial Board. (2016, December 17). Unequal sentences for blacks and whites. The New York Times. Retrieved from https://www.nytimes.com/2016/12/17/opinion/sunday/unequal-sentences-for-blacks-and-whites.html

29   Douglass, F. (1857, august 3). *An address on west India emancipation*.

30   King Jr., M.L. (1963, April 16). *Letter from Birmingham jail*.

31   Malkin, M. (2017, August 2). Procter & Gamble's identity-politics pandering. National Review. Retrieved from http://www.nationalreview.com/article/450073/procter-gambles-liberal-advertising-falls-flat

32   Greenberg, J. (2015, November 23). Trump's pants on fire tweet that blacks killed 81% of white homicide victims. *PolitiFact*. Retrieved from http://www.politifact.com/truth-o-meter/statements/2015/nov/23/donald-trump/trump-tweet-blacks-white-homicide-victims/

33   U.S. Federal Bureau of Investigation. (2016). *2016 Crime in the United States*. Retrieved from https://ucr.fbi.gov/crime-in-the-u.s/2016/crime-in-the-u.s.-2016/tables/expanded-homicide-data-table-3.xls

34   Harriot, M. (2017, October 3). Why we never talk about black-on-black crime: An answer to white America's most pressing question. *The Root*. Retrieved from https://www.theroot.com/why-we-never-talk-about-black-on-black-crime-an-answer-1819092337

35   Kristof, N.D. (2009, July 4). Talk to the Times: Nicholas D. Kristof. *The New York Times*. Retrieved from http://www.nytimes.com/2009/07/06/business/media/06askthetimes.html

36   Hagan, A.S. (2009). Race and city-county consolidation: Black voting participation and municipal elections, 86-93. *Electronic Theses and Dissertations*. Paper 559.

https://doi.org/10.18297/etd/559

37   Louisville Metro Council. (N.D.). *Districts 1-26*. Retrieved from https://louisvilleky.gov/government/metro-council/districts-1-26

38   Claritas. (2017). *Summary data for county: Jefferson* [Data file]. Retrieved from http://www.healthylouisvillemetro.org/index.php?module=DemographicData&controller=index&action=index

39   Sonka, J. (2016, February 14). *Most boards and commissions in Louisville lack required racial and partisan diversity*. Insider Louisville. Retrieved from https://insiderlouisville.com/metro/most-boards-and-commissions-in-louisville-lack-required-ethnic-and-partisan-diversity/

40   The League of Women Voters. (2017). *Felony disenfranchisement in the commonwealth of Kentucky: A report of The League of Women Voters of Kentucky*. Retrieved from https://lwvky.files.wordpress.com/2017/02/kentucky-felony-

disenfranchisement-report-feb-17-final-docx.pdf

41   The League of Women Voters. (2017). *Felony disenfranchisement in the commonwealth of Kentucky: A report of The League of Women Voters of Kentucky.* Retrieved from https://lwvky.files.wordpress.com/2017/02/kentucky-felony-disenfranchisement-report-feb-17-final-docx.pdf

Cummings, S. & Price, M. (1997). Race relations and public policy in Louisville: historical development of an urban underclass. *Journal of Black Studies*, 27(5), 615-p649.

Fosl, Catherine and K'Meyer, Tracy Elaine. (2009). *Freedom on the border: An oral history of the civil rights movement in Kentucky,* 86-93.

Yater, G. H. (2001). Louisville: An historical overview. In J. E. Kleber (Ed.). *The encyclopedia of Louisville,* xv-xxxi. Lexington: The University Press of Kentucky.

42   Collins, W.T. (1869, May 29). *National Memorial Day: A record of ceremonies over the graves of the Union soldiers.*

43   Davis, J. (1861, January 21). *Farewell speech to the U.S. Sentate.*

44   Kentucky Department of Juvenile Justice. (2017). *Kentucky 2017 Updated Plan for Compliance with the Disproportionate Minority Contact Core Requirement.*

45   Dawson-Edwards, C., Tewksbury, R., Higgins, G.E., & Rausch, C. (2014). *Disproportionate Minority Contact in Kentucky: Statewide Assessment Report.*

46   Dawson-Edwards, C., Nelson, N., & Nuss, K. (2017). What's fueling DMC? The role of school discipline decisions on disproportionality in the Juvenile Justice System. In N. Parsons-Pollard (Ed). *Disproportionate Minority Contact.* (2nd ed.). Durham, NC: Carolina Academic Press.

47   Dawson-Edwards, C., Tewksbury, R., Higgins, G.E., & Rausch, C. (2014). *Disproportionate Minority Contact in Kentucky: Statewide Assessment Report.*

48   Restorative Justice Louisville. (2013). *2013 Annual Report.* Retrieved from http://www.rjlou.org/app/webroot/images/RJL-2013-AR.pdf

49   Restorative Justice Louisville. (2017). *Board Report FY 17.*

50   Payne, A.A., & Welch, K. (2015). Restorative justice in schools: The influence of race on restorative discipline. *Youth & Society*, 47, 539-564.

51   Jefferson County Public Schools. (N.D.). Discipline & school climate and culture. *Envision Equity Scorecard.* Retrieved from https://www.jefferson.kyschools.us/sites/default/files/Envision%20Equity%20Scorecard%20Discipline%20School%20Climate%20Culture.pdf

52   Vanderhaar, J.E., Petrosko, J.M., & Munoz, M.A. (2015). Reconsidering the alternatives: The relationship among suspension, placement, subsequent juvenile detention, and the salience of race. In D.J. Losen (Ed.). *Closing the School Discipline Gap: Equitable Remedies for Excessive Exclusion.* Teachers College Press: New York, NY.

53   Dawson-Edwards, C. (2016). Restorative Justice. In W.G. Jennings (Ed). *The Encyclopedia of Crime and Punishment.*

54   TIME Magazine. *The 20 most influential Americans of all time.* Accessible at http://newsfeed.time.com/2012/07/25/the-20-most-influential-americans-of-all-time/slide/all/

55   University of Louisville Center for Environmental Policy and Management. (N.D.). *West Louisville strategies for success.* Retrieved from https://louisville.edu/cepm/westlou/west-louisville-general/vacant-properties-campaign-presentation/

56   Davis, P.C. (1988). Law as Microaggression. *The Yale Law Journal, 98,* 1559, 1576.

57   University of Louisville Center for Environmental Policy and Management. (N.D.). *West Louisville strategies for success.* Retrieved from https://louisville.edu/cepm/westlou/west-louisville-general/vacant-properties-campaign-presentation/

58   Glowicki, M. (2016, December 15). Ruling: Judge Olu Stevens wrong to dismiss jury. The Courier-Journal. Retrieved from https://www.courier-journal.com/story/news/crime/2016/12/15/judges-dismiss-juries-race/95480572/.

59   King Jr., M.L. (1962, September 12). *Forbes.* Retrieved from https://www.forbes.com/quotes/6689/

60   Coates, T. (2014). The case for reparations. *The Atlantic.* Retrieved from https://www.theatlantic.com/magazine/

archive/2014/06/the-case-for-reparations/361631/

61   Thorkelson, B. (2017, Feb. 2). Stay hopeful and do 'uncomfortable things,' advises justice advocate Bryan Stevenson. *Yale University News*. Retrieved from https://news.yale.edu/2017/02/02/stay-hopeful-and-do-uncomfortable-things-advises-justice-advocate-bryan-stevenson

62   Hobbs, H. & Stoops, N. (2002). Demographic trends in the 20th century: Census 2000 special reports. *U.S. Census*. Retrieved from https://www.census.gov/prod/2002pubs/censr-4.pdf

63   Cohn, D., Lopez, M.H., Passel, J. (2011, March 24). Hispanics account for more than half of nation's growth in past decade. *Pew Research Center*. Retrieved from http://www.pewhispanic.org/2011/03/24/hispanics-account-for-more-than-half-of-nations-growth-in-past-decade/

64   Makela, K., Maznevski, M.L., Stahl, G.K., & Zander, L. (2010). A look at the bright side of multicultural team diversity. Scandinavian Journal of Management, 26, 439-447. https://doi.org/10.1016/j.scaman.2010.09.009

65   Jefferson County Public Schools. (2018). Current_enrollment_race_gender_hs [Data file]. 2017-2018 Data Book. Retrieved from https://www.jefferson.kyschools.us/departments/data-management-research/data-books

66   Kentucky School Boards Association. (2015, January 10). *Jefferson County Public Schools: Student demographics: Board orientation*. Retrieved from https://portal.ksba.org/Secure/Login.aspx?ReturnUrl=%2fSecure%2fErrors.aspx%3faspxerrorpath%3d%2fpublic%2fMeeting%2fAttachments%2fDisplayAttachment.aspx&aspxerrorpath=/public/Meeting/Attachments/DisplayAttachment.aspx

67   Kentucky Commission on Human Rights. (2008). *An overview of the minority educators in Kentucky's public schools.* Retrieved from https://kchr.ky.gov/reports/Documents/Reports/MinorityEducatorsinKY.pdf

68   Kentucky Commission on Human Rights. (2009). *The state of African Americans minority in Kentucky.* Retrieved from https://kchr.ky.gov/reports/Documents/Reports/WhitePaperRevised.pdf

69   Kentucky Department of Education. (2017, May 2). *Kentucky education facts*. Retrieved from https://education.ky.gov/comm/edfacts/Pages/default.aspx

70   Jefferson County Public Schools. (2018). Suspensions_by_race_gender_hs [Data file]. *2017-2018 Data Book.* Retrieved from https://www.jefferson.kyschools.us/departments/data-management-research/data-books

71   Great Schools Partnership. (2013, September 3). Opportunity gap. *Glossary of Education Reform.* Retrieved from http://edglossary.org/opportunity-gap/

72   Kentucky Department of Education. (2017, October 13). *School report card: Jefferson County, 2016-17.* Retrieved from http://applications.education.ky.gov/src/ProfileByDistrict.aspx

73   Integrated Post Secondary Education Data System. (N.D.). Degree completions [Data file]. *55,000 Degrees Education Data Dashboard.* Retrieved from http://dashboard.55000degrees.org/postsecondary/degree-%20completions/

74   Bureau of Labor Statistics. (2016, May 11). *Weekly earnings by educational attainment in first quarter 2016.* Retrieved from https://www.bls.gov/opub/ted/2016/weekly-earnings-by-educational-attainment-in-first-quarter-2016.htm

75   U.S. Department of Health & Human Services, Administration for Children and Families, Administration on Children, Youth and Families, Children's Bureau. (2016). *Child maltreatment 2014.* Retrieved from http://www.acf.hhs.gov/programs/cb/research-data-technology/statistics-research/child-maltreatment

76   Johnson, A. (2016, November 17). *Forum to address racial disproportionality and disparities for children of color.* Race Community and Child Welfare Initiative and Kentucky Cabinet for Health and Family Services, Department for Community Based Services. Muhammad Ali Center, Louisville: KY.

77   U.S. Department for Health and Human Services, Administration for Children and Families, Administration on Children Youth and Families, Children's Bureau. (July, 2017). *Child welfare outcomes 2010-2014: Report to Congress.* Retrieved from https://www.acf.hhs.gov/cb/resource/cwo-10-14.

78   Clifford, S. & Silver-Greenberg, J. (2017, July 21). Foster care as punishment: The new reality of 'jane crow". *The New York Times.* Retrieved from https://www.nytimes.com/2017/07/21/nyregion/foster-care-nyc-jane-crow.html?rref=collection%2Ftimestopic%2FAdministration%20for%20Children%27s%20Services&action=click&contentCollection=timestopics&region=stream&module=stream_unit&version=latest&contentPlacement=5&pgtype=collection

79   Johnson, L., Antle, B. F., & Barbee, A. P. (2009). Addressing disproportionality and disparity in child welfare:

Evaluation of an anti-racism training for community service providers. *Children and Youth Services Review*. *31*, 688-696.

80   Barbee, A. P., Henry, K., & Johnson, L. (2010). Report on Undoing Racism: Evaluation and impact of RCCW. University of Louisville, Louisville: KY.

81   Kentucky Commission on Human Rights. (2009). *The state of African Americans in Kentucky*. Louisville: KY.

82   Goode, R.W. (2016, January 29). Reframing the narrative around black men. *Black Enterprise*. Retrieved from http://www.blackenterprise.com/reframing-the-narrative-around-black-men/

83   Integrated Public Use Microdata Series-USA. (2016). *U.S. Census data for social, economic, and health research: Louisville data studio analysis, 2012-2016*. Retrieved from https://usa.ipums.org/usa/

84   U.S. Census Bureau. (2016, February 23). *Survey of business owners (SBO) – Survey results: 2012*. Retrieved from https://www.census.gov/library/publications/2012/econ/2012-sbo.html

85   Pruitt, S.L. (2016, July 18). *Courage in the face of change*. Kentucky Department of Education. Accessisble at https://education.ky.gov/CommOfEd/blog/Documents/071816%20Courage%20for%20change.pdf

86   Baldwin, J. (1963, December 21). A talk to teachers. *The Saturday Review*.

87   Harris, C. I. (1993). Whiteness as property. *Harvard Law Review*, 1707-1791.

88   Perry, T., Steele, C., & Hilliard, A. G. (2003). *Young, gifted, and black: Promoting high achievement among African-American students*. Boston, MA: Beacon Press.

89   Woodson, C. G. (1933). *The mis-education of the Negro*. Trenton, NJ: First Africa World Press.

90   Anderson, C. (2016). *White rage: The unspoken truth of our racial divide*. New York, NY: Bloomsbury.

91   Larimer, S. (2018). 'Kids are freezing': Amid bitter cold, Baltimore schools, students struggle. *The Washington Post*. Retrieved from https://www.washingtonpost.com/local/education/kids-are-freezing-amid-bitter-cold-baltimore-schools-students-struggle/2018/01/05/8c213eec-f183-11e7-b390-a36dc3fa2842_story.html?utm_term=.4d8c217c53ea

92   Anderson, J. (2017). State opens $35 million youth detention facility in Baltimore. *The Baltimore Sun*. Retrieved from http://www.baltimoresun.com/news/maryland/crime/bs-md-ci-new-youth-jail-20170907-story.html

93   Colthrop, J. (2016). Detroit teacher says sick-outs are in response to 'deplorable' conditions at DPS schools. *Click on Detroit*. Retrieved from https://www.clickondetroit.com/news/detroit-teacher-says-sick-outs-are-in-response-to-deplorable-conditions-at-dps-schools

94   Kozol, J. (1991). *Savage inequalities: Children in America's schools*. New York, NY: Broadway Paperbacks.

95   Crenshaw, K., Ocen, P., & Nanda, J. (2015). *Black girls matter: Pushed out, overpoliced, and underprotected*. Center for Intersectionality and Social Policy Studies, Columbia University.

96   Dumas, M. J. (2016). Against the dark: Antiblackness in education policy and discourse. *Theory Into Practice, 55* (1), 11-19.

97   U.S. Department of Education. (2016). Office of Planning, Evaluation and Policy Development, Policy and Program Studies Service. *The State of Racial Diversity in the Educator Workforce*, Washington, D.C.

98   Jefferson County Public School System. (2017). *Opportunity, Data, Development, and Systems Report*.

99   Bridgeland, J., & Bruce, M. (2011). 2011 National Survey of School Counselors: Counseling at a Crossroads. *College Board Advocacy & Policy Center*.

100 Jefferson County Public School System. (2017). *Opportunity, Data, Development, and Systems Report*.

101 Gershenson, S., Hart, C., Lindsay, C. A., & Papageorge, N. W. (2017). The long-run impacts of same-race teachers (No. 10630). *Institute for the Study of Labor (IZA)*.

102 Lindsay, C. A. & Hart, C. M. D. (2017). Teacher race and school discipline: Are students suspended less often when they have a teacher of the same race? *Education Next*. Retrieved from http://educationnext.org/teacher-race-and-school-discipline-suspensions-research/

103 Chandler, P. T. (2009). Blinded by the white: Social studies and raceless pedagogies. *The Journal of Educational Thoughts (JET)/Revue de la Pensée Educative*, 259-288.

104 Morrison, T. (1992). Playing in the dark: Whiteness and the literary imagination. Vintage Books.

105 Baldwin, J. (1963). A talk to teachers. *The Saturday Review*.

106 Perry, T., Steele, C., & Hilliard, A. G. (2003). *Young, gifted, and Black: Promoting high achievement among African-American students*. Boston, MA: Beacon Press.

107 Golding, S. (2017). Florida high school students stage sit in to demand African American history to be taught year round. *Vibe*. Retrieved from https://www.vibe.com/2017/01/florida-student-demonstration-

african-american-history/

108 Nobles, W. (1998). Foreword. In A. G. Hilliard, *SBA: The reawakening of the African mind*. Makare Pub Co.

109 Jefferson County Public School System. (2017). JCPS Data Books, 2017-2018: Suspensions by Race and Gender. Retrieved from https://www.jefferson.kyschools.us/sites/default/files/jcpsdbk258.pdf

110 Skiba, R. J., & Williams, N. T. (2014). Are Black kids worse? Myths and facts about racial differences in behavior. *The Equity Project at Indiana University*.

111 King, Jr, M. L. (1963). Letter from Birmingham city jail.

112 Shakur, A. (1987). Assata: An Autobiography. Chicago, IL: Zed Books.

113 55,000 Degrees Education Data Dashboard. (N.D.). *JCPS college going by race/ethnicity or sex* [Data file]. Retrieved from http://dashboard.55000degrees.org/college-transition/college-going/

114 55,000 Degrees Education Data Dashboard. (N.D.). *JCPS college going by race/ethnicity or sex* [Data file]. Retrieved from http://dashboard.55000degrees.org/college-transition/college-going/

115 55,000 Degrees Education Data Dashboard. (N.D.). *JCPS graduation rates* [Data file]. Retrieved from http://dashboard.55000degrees.org/high-school/jcps-graduation-rates/

116 55,000 Degrees Education Data Dashboard. (N.D.). *Jefferson County Public Schools college and career readiness with demographic breakdown* [Data file]. Retrieved from http://dashboard.55000degrees.org/high-school/college-career-readiness/

117 55,000 Degrees Education Data Dashboard. (N.D.). *Education attainment by race, age, and sex* [Data file]. Retrieved from http://dashboard.55000degrees.org/community/education-attainment-of-working-age-population/

118 Carnevale, A.P., Smith, N., & Strohl, J. (2013). Recovery: Job growth and education requirements through 2020. *Georgetown University Center on Education and the Workforce*. Retrieved from https://cew.georgetown.edu/wp-content/uploads/2014/11/Recovery2020.ES_.Web_.pdf

119 55,000 Degrees. (2015). *Fast Forward 2015 Report*. Retrieved from http://www.55000degrees.org/wp-content/uploads/2015/12/2015-Fast-Forward-Report.pdf

120 County Health Rankings & Roadmaps. (2017). *Children in poverty: Percentage of children under 18 in poverty*. Retrieved from http://www.countyhealthrankings.org/app/kentucky/2017/measure/factors/24/data

121 55,000 Degrees Education Data Dashboard. (N.D.). *Local postsecondary graduation rates by institution, sector, and race* [Data file]. Retrieved from http://dashboard.55000degrees.org/postsecondary/graduation-rates/

122 Kentucky Council on Postsecondary Education. (N.D.). *Kentucky public postsecondary institutions: Annual tuition and mandatory fees for full-time undergraduate students*. Retrieved from http://cpe.ky.gov/data/reports/TuitionandFeesPublicFTUndergrad200616.pdf

123 Jefferson County Public Schools. (2018*)*. Current_enrollment_race_gender_hs *[Data file]. 2017-2018 Data Book*. Retrieved from https://www.jefferson.kyschools.us/departments/data-management-research/data-books

124 Jefferson County Public Schools. (2018). Gap_read_math_hs [Data file]. *2017-2018 Data Book*. Retrieved from https://www.jefferson.kyschools.us/about/accountability/equity

125 JCPS Race and Equity Policy Committee. (2017, October 11). *Programmatic access*. Retrieved from https://portal.ksba.org/public/Agency.aspx?PublicAgencyID=89&AgencyTypeID=1 iiisang d from cess. Policy Committe.ndbook. n HandSnt heating it up. It takes time to learn how to cook things taht et and I ju

126 Jefferson County Public Schools. (2017). *Student support and behavior intervention handbook*. Retrieved from https://www.jefferson.kyschools.us/sites/default/files/forms/Student%20Support%20and%20Behavior%20Intervention%20Handbook.pdf

127 Heckman, J.J. (2016). *There's more to gain by taking a comprehensive approach to early childhood development.* Retrieved from https://heckmanequation.org/assets/2017/01/F_Heckman_CBAOnePager_120516.pdf

128 Center for Health Equity. (2017). 2017 Health equity report: Uncovering the root causes of health. *Louisville Metro Department of Public Health and Wellness.* Retrieved from https://louisvilleky.gov/government/center-health-equity/health-equity-report

129 Centers for Disease Control and Prevention. (2010). 500 cities project: Local data for better health [Data file]. Retrieved from https://nccd.cdc.gov/500_Cities/rdPage.aspx?rdReport=DPH_500_Cities.InteractiveMap&islCategories=HLTHOUT&islMeasures=ARTHRITIS&islStates=59&rdRnd=18473

130 Center for Health Equity. (2014). Louisville Metro Health Equity Report. *Department of Public Health and Wellness.* Retrieved from https://louisvilleky.gov/sites/default/files/health_and_wellness/che/health_equity_report/her2014_7_31_14.pdf

131 City-Data. (2013). *Louisville, Kentucky (KY) poverty rate data* [Data file]. Retrieved fromhttp://www.city-data.com/poverty/poverty-Louisville-Kentucky.html

132 Center for Health Equity. (2014). Louisville Metro Health Equity Report. *Department of Public Health and Wellness.* Retrieved from https://louisvilleky.gov/sites/default/files/health_and_wellness/che/health_equity_report/her2014_7_31_14.pdf

133 Center for Health Equity. (2014). Louisville Metro Health Equity Report. *Department of Public Health and Wellness.* Retrieved from https://louisvilleky.gov/sites/default/files/health_and_wellness/che/health_equity_report/her2014_7_31_14.pdf

134 Healthy Start. (2017). Louisville Metro Department of Public Health and Wellness. Retrieved from https://louisvilleky.gov/government/health-wellness/healthy-start

135 Center for Health Equity. (2014). Louisville Metro Health Equity Report. *Department of Public Health and Wellness.* Retrieved from https://louisvilleky.gov/sites/default/files/health_and_wellness/che/health_equity_report/her2014_7_31_14.pdf

136 Gillespie, L. (2017, March 3). *New data show stark health disparities in East, West Louisville.* WFPL News Louisville. Retrieved from http://wfpl.org/new-data-show-stark-health-disparities-east-west-louisville/

137 Obama, B. (2017, August 12). Twitter.

138 Community Farm Alliance. (2007). *Bridging the divide: Growing self-sufficiency in our food supply.* Retrieved from http://cfaky.org/test/wp-content/uploads/2015/03/BridgingTheDivide.pdf

139 Center for Health Equity. (2017). *Louisville Metro Health Equity Report 2017.* Louisville, KY: Louisville Metro Public Health and Wellness.

140 The Sentencing Project. (2017). *Trends in U.S. Corrections* [Data file]. Retrieved from https://sentencingproject.org/wp-content/uploads/2016/01/Trends-in-US-Corrections.pdf

141 U.S. Census Bureau. (2015). *2009-2013 5-year American Community Survey.* Retrieved from https://www.census.gov/programs-surveys/acs/about.html

142 Kentucky Department of Corrections. *Research and Statistics.* Retrieved from https://corrections.ky.gov/about/Pages/ResearchandStatistics.aspx

143 The Sentencing Project. (2013). *Shadow Report to the United Nations on Racial Disparities in the United States Criminal Justice System.* Retrieved from http://www.sentencingproject.org/publications/shadow-report-to-the-united-nations-human-rights-committee-regarding-racial-disparities-in-the-united-states-criminal-justice-system/

144 Louisville Metro Police Department Homicide Unit

145 McAfee, M. (May 2017). Convening address to civic and educational leaders. *By All Means, Harvard University.*

146 Louisville Metro Police Department Homicide Unit

147 Desrochers, D. (2017, June 28). 3-day limit on painkiller prescriptions among new laws taking effect Thursday. *Lexington Herald-Leader.* Retrieved from http://www.kentucky.com/news/politics-government/article158710024.html

148 Kentucky Commission on Human Rights. (2010). *Status of African Americans in Kentucky: 2010 Revised Edition.* Retrieved from https://kchr.ky.gov/reports/Documents/Reports/AAStatus2010.pdf

149 Cherry, R. (2017, February 16). *Race and rising violent crime*. RealClearPolicy. Retrived from http://www. realclearpolicy.com/articles/2017/02/16/race_and_rising_violent_crime.html

150 Herrman, H., Saxena, S., Moodie, M. (Eds.). (2005). *Promoting mental health: Concepts, emerging evidence, practice: Report of the World Health Organization, Department of Mental Health and Substance Abuse in collaboration with the Victorian Health Promotion Foundation and the University of Melbourne* (pp. XVIII). Geneva: WHO. Retrieved from http://www.who.int/mental_health/evidence/MH_Promotion_Book.pdf

151 World Health Organization. (2017). *Depression and other common mental disorders: Global health estimates*. WHO/MSD/MER/2017.2 Geneva: WHO. Retrieved from http://www.who.int/mental_health/management/depression/prevalence_global_health_estimates/en/

152 Pearson, G., Hines-Martin, V., Evan, L., York, J., Kane, C., & Yearwood, E. (2015). Addressing gaps in mental health needs of diverse, at-risk, underserved, and disenfranchised populations: A call for nursing action. *Archives of Psychiatric Nursing,* 29 (2015) 14–18.

153 Pearson, G., Evans, L., Hines-Martin, V., Yearwood, E., York, J. & Kane, C. (2014). Promoting the mental health of families. *Nursing Outlook*, 62 (3), 225 – 227.

154 Fischer, G. (2017, July 6). *Capturing Ali's spirit: Creating a city of peace and safety.* City of Louisville, Kentucky. Retrieved from https://louisvilleky.gov/news/mayor-fischers-remarks-capturing-alis-spirit-creating-city-peace-and-safety

155 City of Louisville, Kentucky. (N.D.). *Louisville Affordable Housing Trust Fund*. Retrieved from https://louisvilleky.gov/government/housing-community-development/louisville-affordable-housing-trust-fund

156 U.S. Census Bureau. (2016). *2011-2015 American Community Survey 5 Year Estimate*. Retrieved from https://factfinder.census.gov/.

157 Mazza, C., & Perry, A. (2017). *Fatherhood in America: Social work perspectives on a changing society.* Springfield, IL: Charles C. Thomas Publishers.

158 Mazza, C., & Perry, A. (2017). *Fatherhood in America: Social work perspectives on a changing society.* Springfield, IL: Charles C. Thomas Publishers.

159 Adler, M.A., & Lenz, K. (2017). *Father involvement in the early years: An international comparison of policy and practice.* Bristol, United Kingdom: Policy Press.

160 Adler, M.A., & Lenz, K. (2017). *Father involvement in the early years: An international comparison of policy and practice.* Bristol, United Kingdom: Policy Press.

161 National Fair Housing Alliance. (2017, April 19). *New report makes 'the case for fair housing' as segregation persists & hate crimes rise.* Retrieved from http://nationalfairhousing.org/2017/04/19/new-report-makes-the-case-for-fair-housing-as-segregation-persists-hate-crimes-rise/

162 The Fair Housing Center of Greater Boston. (N.D.) *1948-1968: Unenforceable restrictive covenants.* Retrieved from http://www.bostonfairhousing.org/timeline/1948-1968-Unenforceable-Restrictive-Covenants.html

163 Frohlich, T. C. & Kent, A. (2015, August 19). America's most segregated cities. *24/7 Wall St.* Retrieved from http://247wallst.com/special-report/2015/08/19/americas-most-segregated-cities/3/

164 Jefferson County Public Schools. (2018). Homeless_demographic_hs [Data file]. *2017-2018 Data Book.* Retrieved from https://www.jefferson.kyschools.us/departments/data-management-research/data-books

165 Leighton, G.R. (1937). Louisville, Kentucky: An American museum piece. *Harper's Magazine.* Retrieved from https://harpers.org/archive/1937/09/louisville-kentucky/

166 Home Owner's Loan Corporation Division of Research and Statistics. (1937, September 22). *Explanation text.* Retrieved from https://lojic.maps.arcgis.com/apps/MapSeries/index.html?appid=e4d29907953c4094a17cb9ea8f8f89de

167 U.S. Census. (2010). *Summary file 1.* Retrieved from https://www.census.gov/newsroom/releases/archives/2010_census/cb11-cn165.html

168 U.S. Census. (2010). *Summary file 1.* Retrieved from https://www.census.gov/newsroom/releases/archives/2010_census/cb11-cn165.html

169 The American City Planning Institute. (1918). *Title of document?* (pp. 44 -45). City, State: Publisher.

170 Freund, D. (2007). *Colored property: State policy and white racial politics in suburban America (*pp. 73-74). Chicago, IL:

University of Chicago Press.

171 Harlan Bartholomew and Associates. (1932). *The Negro Housing Problem in Louisville*. St. Louis, MO: Washington University Archives.

172 Harlan Bartholomew and Associates. (1932). *The Negro Housing Problem in Louisville*. St. Louis, MO: Washington University Archives.

173 Harlan Bartholomew and Associates. (1932). *The Negro Housing Problem in Louisville*. St. Louis, MO: Washington University Archives.

174 Housing & Community Development. (2016, October 26). *Louisville CARES Fact Sheet*. Retrieved from https://louisvilleky.gov/sites/default/files/housing_community_development/lou_cares_fact_sheet_final_10-26-16.pdf

175 Barbour, S. (2016, November 15). Angela Davis speech in Louisville 11-15-2016 [Audio file]. *SoundCloud*. Retrived from https://soundcloud.com/johnsdoemain/angela-davis-speech-in-louisville-11-15-2016

176 Burton, D.O. & Barnes, Brian C.B. (2017, January 3). Shifting philanthropy from charity to justice. *Stanford Social Innovation Review*. Retrieved from https://ssir.org/articles/entry/shifting_philanthropy_from_charity_to_justice

177 City of Louisville, Kentucky. (2017). *Property Reports*. Retrieved from http://portal.louisvilleky.gov/codesandregs/property-reports/vacantstructures

178 Bush, B. (2016, September 6). Plan transforms 'neighborhood watch.' *The Courier-Journal*. Retrieved from https://www.courier-journal.com/story/opinion/columnists/2016/09/06/bridget-bush-plan-transforms-neighborhood-watch/89736798/

179 U.S. Department of Housing and Urban Development. (N.D.). *Affirmatively Furthering Fair Housing (AFFH)*. Retrieved from https://www.hudexchange.info/programs/affh/

180 U.S. Census Bureau. (2015). *2010-2014 5-year American Community Survey*. Retrieved from https://www.census.gov/programs-surveys/acs/about.html

181 Rothstein, R. (2017). *The Color of Law: A Forgotten History of How Our Government Segregated America*. New York, NY: Liveright.

182 Kentucky Department of Corrections. *Research and Statistics*. Retrieved from https://corrections.ky.gov/about/Pages/ResearchandStatistics.aspx

183 The Sentencing Project. (2013). *Shadow Report to the United Nations on Racial Disparities in the United States Criminal Justice System*. Retrieved from http://www.sentencingproject.org/publications/shadow-report-to-the-united-nations-human-rights-committee-regarding-racial-disparities-in-the-united-states-criminal-justice-system/

184 Pew Research Center. (2013). *Incarceration gap widens between whites and blacks*. Retrieved from http://www.pewresearch.org/fact-tank/2013/09/06/incarceration-gap-between-whites-and-blacks-widens/

185 Metropolitan Housing Coalition, University of Louisville Center for Envrionmental Policy & Management. (2017, December 12). *2017 State of metropolitan housing report*. Retrieved from http://www.metropolitanhousing.org/wp-content/uploads/member_docs/2017SMHR_FINAL_Web.pdf

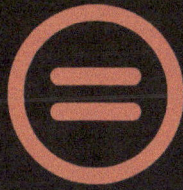

Louisville Urban League

Join the Movement!

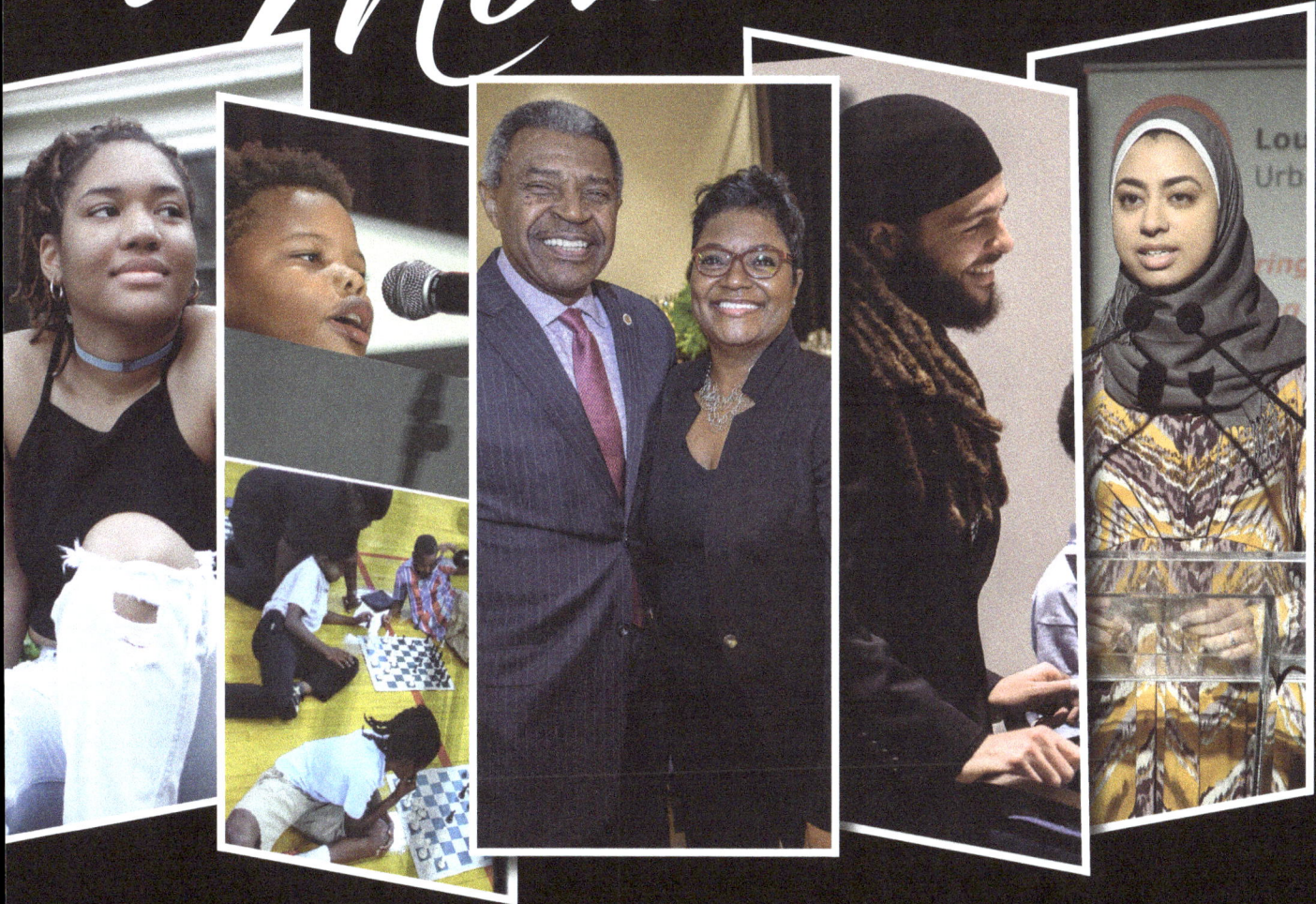

JOBS · JUSTICE · EDUCATION · HEALTH · HOUSING

Louisville Urban League I 1535 W Broadway I Louisville, KY 40203 I (502) 585-4622

www.LUL.org